WORKBOOK TO ACCOMPANY

MOSBY'S
CANADIAN
TEXTBOOK
FOR THE
SUPPORT
WORKER

FOURTH CANADIAN EDITION

Sheila A. Sorrentino RN, PhD
Curriculum and Health Care Consultant
Anthem, Arizona

Leighann N. Remmert RN, MS
Health Occupations Instructor, Lincolnland Technical Education
Center
Lincoln, Illinois

Relda T. Kelly RN, MSN
Professor Emeritus, Kankakee Community College
Kankakee, Illinois
Parish Nurse, Wesley United Methodist Church
Bradley, Illinois

Canadian Authors

Mary J. Wilk RN, GNC(C), BA, BScN, MN
Professor and Coordinator, Personal Support Worker Program,
Fanshawe College, London, Ontario

Mary Cammaert RN
Coordinator, Personal Support Worker Program, Fanshawe College,
St. Thomas Elgin Campus, London, Ontario

ELSEVIER

ELSEVIER

Copyright © 2018 Elsevier Canada, a division of Reed Elsevier Canada, Ltd.

Adapted from *Workbook to Accompany Mosby's Canadian Textbook for the Support Worker*, 3rd Canadian edition, rev. reprint by Relda T. Kelly, Sheila A. Sorrentino, Leighann N. Remmert, Mary J. Wilk, and Deborah Schuh. Copyright © 2013 (ISBN: 978-1-92740-658-8). Previous editions copyrighted 2013, 2009.

All rights reserved. No part of this publication may be reproduced or transmitted in any form or by any means, electronic or mechanical, including photocopy, recording, or any information storage and retrieval system, without permission in writing from the publisher. Reproducing passages from this book without such written permission is an infringement of copyright law.

Requests for permission to make copies of any part of the work should be mailed to: College Licensing Officer, access ©, 1 Yonge Street, Suite 1900, Toronto, ON, M5E 1E5. Fax: (416) 868-1621. All other inquiries should be directed to the publisher.

Every reasonable effort has been made to acquire permission for copyrighted material used in this text and to acknowledge all such indebtedness accurately. Any errors and omissions called to the publisher's attention will be corrected in future printings.

NOTICES

Knowledge and best practice in this field are constantly changing. As new research and experience broaden our understanding, changes in research methods, professional practices, or medical treatment may become necessary.

Practitioners and researchers must always rely on their own experience and knowledge in evaluating and using any information, methods, compounds, or experiments described herein. In using such information or methods, they should be mindful of their own safety and the safety of others, including parties for whom they have a professional responsibility.

With respect to any drug or pharmaceutical products identified, readers are advised to check the most current information provided (i) on procedures featured or (ii) by the manufacturer of each product to be administered to verify the recommended dose or formula, the method and duration of administration, and the contraindications. It is the responsibility of practitioners, relying on their own experience and knowledge of their patients, to make diagnoses, to determine dosages and the best treatment for each individual patient, and to take all appropriate safety precautions.

To the fullest extent of the law, neither the Publisher nor the authors, contributors, or editors assume any liability for any injury and/or damage to persons or property as a matter of products liability, negligence, or otherwise, or from any use or operation of any methods, products, instructions, or ideas contained in the material herein.

The Publisher

Library and Archives Canada Cataloguing in Publication

Sorrentino, Sheila A., author
  Workbook to accompany Mosby's Canadian textbook
for the support worker / Sheila A. Sorrentino RN, PhD (Curriculum
and Health Care Consultant, Anthem, Arizona), Leighann N. Remmert
RN, MS (Health Occupations Instructor, Lincolnland Technical
Education Center, Lincoln, Illinois), Relda T. Kelly RN, MSN (Professor
Emeritus, Kankakee Community College, Kankakee, Illinois; Parish
Nurse, Wesley United Methodist Church, Bradley, Illinois) ; Canadian
authors, Mary J. Wilk RN, GNC(C), BA, BScN, MN (Professor and
Coordinator, Personal Support Program, Fanshawe College,
London, Ontario), Mary Cammert, RN (Coordinator Personal Support
Worker Program, Fanshawe College, St. Thomas Elgin Campus, London,
Ontario). – Fourth Canadian edition.

Supplement to: Mosby's Canadian textbook for the support worker.
ISBN 978-1-77172-043-4 (paperback)

  1. Nurses' aides—Problems, exercises, etc. 2. Care of the sick—Problems, exercises, etc. I. Kelly, Relda Timmeney, author II. Wilk, Mary J., author III. Remmert, Leighann N., author IV. Cammaert, Mary, author V. Title.

RT84.S67 2017 Suppl.   610.7306'98   C2016-906296-1

ISBN 978-1-77172-127-1 (paperback)

Vice President, Publishing: Ann Millar
Content Strategist (Acquisitions): Roberta A. Spinosa-Millman
Content Development Specialist: Sandy Matos
Publishing Services Manager: Jeff Patterson
Senior Project Manager: Tracey Schriefer

Copy Editor: Sherry Hinman
Proofreader: Anne Ostroff
Cover: Muthukumaran Thangaraj
Typesetting and Assembly: TnQ

Elsevier Canada
555 Richmond Street West, Suite 1100, Toronto, ON, Canada M5V 3B1
Phone: 1-866-896-3331
Fax: 1-855-215-5738

7 8 9 23 22 21

Ebook ISBN: 978-1-77172-129-5

 Working together to grow libraries in developing countries

www.elsevier.com • www.bookaid.org

Contents

Copyright © 2018 Elsevier Canada, a division of Reed Elsevier Canada, Ltd.

Copyright © 2018 Elsevier Canada, a division of Reed Elsevier Canada, Ltd.

Introduction

This workbook is intended to be used with *Mosby's Canadian Textbook for the Support Worker*, Fourth Canadian Edition. Additional resources are not required to complete the workbook exercises.

This workbook is designed as a study guide to help you apply what you have learned in each chapter of the textbook. As a supplement to this workbook, procedure checklists are featured on the Evolve website for *Mosby's Canadian Textbook for the Support Worker*, Fourth Canadian Edition. These checklists are designed to help you become more skilled at performing procedures to enhance the quality of care. Consult with your instructor for correct answers to material presented in this workbook and on the Evolve website's procedure checklists. The Evolve website for *Mosby's Canadian Textbook for the Support Worker*, Fourth Canadian Edition, can be accessed at http://evolve.elsevier.com/Canada/Sorrentino/SupportWorker.

As a support worker, you are an important member of the health care team. Completing the exercises in this workbook will increase your knowledge and skills. Our goal is to prepare you to provide the best possible care to your clients and to encourage you to take pride in a job well done.

The Role of the Support Worker

TRUE OR FALSE

Circle T for true, or circle F for false.

1. **T F** Most adults over the age of 70 years have a disabling illness.

2. **T F** Support workers are expected to adapt their work to the setting and needs of the client.

3. **T F** Unregulated care providers must adhere to their employer's code of behaviour at all times.

4. **T F** Discretion means keeping all private information to yourself.

5. **T F** It is okay to discuss your personal problems with a client you have been working with for a long time.

6. **T F** The goal of support workers is to demonstrate true compassionate care for their clients and families at all times.

7. **T F** Wearing any amount of fragrance can cause breathing problems for some clients.

8. **T F** In long-term care facilities, support workers assist clients with complex health challenges.

MULTIPLE RESPONSE

From the list below, choose all of the correct answers.

9. Activities of daily living include:
   A. Bathing
   B. Toileting
   C. Feeding
   D. Personal hygiene
   E. Ambulating or transferring
   F. Preparing meals

Copyright © 2018 Elsevier Canada, a division of Reed Elsevier Canada, Ltd.

10. Support workers' responsibilities can be grouped into the following categories:
    A. Personal care
    B. Assessing and treating physical challenges
    C. Financial support
    D. Family support
    E. Legal assistance
    F. Social support
    G. Support for nurses and other professionals
    H. Housekeeping/home management

11. Which statements about support work are correct?
    A. Support work is a regulated profession.
    B. The ultimate goal of support work is to improve the person's quality of life.
    C. Support work services provided to people in their homes help them remain independent and with their families.
    D. Support work makes a difference in people's lives.
    E. Support work requires showing kindness, sensitivity, and understanding to clients.

12. The letters in the acronym *DIPPS* stand for:
    A. Identification
    B. Privacy
    C. Sincerity
    D. Preferences
    E. Discretion
    F. Personal space
    G. Independence
    H. Safety
    I. Dignity

13. To be a true professional, you should demonstrate:
    A. A positive attitude
    B. A sense of responsibility
    C. A professional appearance
    D. Discretion about client information
    E. Discretion about personal matters
    F. Acceptable speech and language
    G. That you engage in lifelong learning

14. Practices for a professional appearance include:
    A. Following dress code policies
    B. Keeping fingernails clean and freshly polished
    C. Wearing clean stockings or socks
    D. Wearing comfortable, clean shoes
    E. Ensuring underclothing cannot be seen or detected
    F. Refraining from wearing makeup
    G. Keeping hair away from the face and off the collar
    H. Wearing mildly scented perfumes, colognes, or aftershaves
    I. Wearing a clean, well-fitting, modest uniform
    J. Wearing an appropriate identification badge

15. When solving problems, which of the following should you consider?
    A. Personal desire to solve the problem
    B. Priorities of support work
    C. Client's viewpoint
    D. Supervisor's viewpoint
    E. Scope of practice
    F. Whether you will be paid extra for solving the problem

16. Where should you find information about your scope of practice?
    A. Clients
    B. Your supervisor
    C. Employer's policies
    D. Friends and co-workers
    E. The educational program

Copyright © 2018 Elsevier Canada, a division of Reed Elsevier Canada, Ltd.

17. The clients you support can be grouped according to their problems, needs, and ages. Some of these groups are:
    A. Healthy older adults who live independently
    B. Mothers and newborns
    C. People with disabilities
    D. People who are in jail
    E. People with medical problems
    F. Athletes receiving therapy for sports injuries
    G. People with mental health problems
    H. People needing rehabilitation
    I. Children
    J. Older adults living in an assisted-living facility
    K. People having surgery

MULTIPLE CHOICE

Circle the best answer.

18. A reflective practice review is:
    A. Thinking about problems that occurred with a co-worker
    B. Being discreet when speaking with a client's family
    C. An honest self-evaluation of all the care you provided to the client
    D. Planning client care around staff availability

19. A support worker is considered to be:
    A. An unregulated care provider
    B. An unregulated nurse
    C. A certified support worker
    D. A regulated care provider

20. A support worker's scope of practice refers to the:
    A. Skills that the employer wants performed
    B. Amount of practice that is needed to perform a skill safely
    C. Legal extent of the role of a support worker
    D. Amount of time it takes to perform a skill

21. Support workers can advocate for their clients by:
    A. Never leaving their clients' side.
    B. Providing empathetic care
    C. Acting appropriately at all times
    D. Speaking or acting on behalf of the client when necessary

22. The ultimate goal of support work is to:
    A. Alleviate the client's pain
    B. Improve the client's quality of life by providing compassionate care
    C. Ensure the client is clean and dry at all times
    D. Perform all assigned duties

23. An example of discretion would be:
    A. Using responsible judgement when speaking about a client
    B. Refraining from using clients' names when talking about them in the lunchroom
    C. Speaking to the client's family and friends about the care the client receives
    D. Talking to your co-worker about your private life while you are making beds

24. Amy is a support worker who has just graduated from school. She plans to wear her engagement ring to work once she is hired. What should you advise her about this?
    A. She will never get a job if she wears her ring.
    B. She has only a small diamond in her ring, so it would be okay to wear it.
    C. She should not wear it around her supervisor.
    D. Her ring can scratch a client and may create an infection control risk, so she should not wear it.

Copyright © 2018 Elsevier Canada, a division of Reed Elsevier Canada, Ltd.

25. Having concern for a client is:
    A. Caring
    B. Sympathy
    C. Enthusiasm
    D. Admiration

26. A way to preserve the client's dignity would be to:
    A. Be considerate
    B. Demonstrate empathy
    C. Be respectful of the client's wishes
    D. Maintain a cheerful approach at all times

27. Understanding your own feelings, strengths, and weaknesses is defined as:
    A. Consideration
    B. Trustworthiness
    C. Conscientiousness
    D. Self-awareness

28. Which is an example of an instrumental activity of daily living (IADL)?
    A. Grooming and dressing
    B. Management of medication
    C. Assisting with meals
    D. Promoting physical comfort

MATCHING

Match each statement in the left column with the correct word in the right column.

29. Supervises LPNs/RPNs and support workers

30. Diagnoses and treats diseases and injuries

31. Provides respiratory treatments and therapies

32. Assesses and plans for nutritional needs

33. Assists people with musculo-skeletal problems

34. Assists people with learning or retaining skills needed to perform activities of daily living

35. Treats people with speech, voice, hearing, communication, or swallowing disorders

36. Assists people with their spiritual needs

37. Helps clients and families with social and emotional issues affecting illness and recovery

A. Occupational therapist

B. Speech–language pathologist

C. Social worker

D. Dietitian

E. Physician

F. Physiotherapist

G. Respiratory therapist

H. Spiritual advisor

I. Nurse

FILL IN THE BLANKS

Complete the following fill-in-the-blank questions in the space provided.

38. A person receiving care in a hospital is called a _____; in a residential facility is called a _____; in the community is called a _____.

Copyright © 2018 Elsevier Canada, a division of Reed Elsevier Canada, Ltd.

The Canadian Health Care System

TRUE OR FALSE

Circle T for true, or circle F for false.

1. **T   F**   Health care service delivery to First Nations and Aboriginal peoples is a provincial or territorial responsibility only.

2. **T   F**   The Canadian health care system has seen a shift in focus from home care to hospital care.

3. **T   F**   Clients are being sent home sooner after hospital procedures.

4. **T   F**   Home care enables some clients to maintain their health and independence.

5. **T   F**   Every province and territory provides primary, secondary, and tertiary health care.

6. **T   F**   Income and social status do not have an influence on health.

7. **T   F**   People can lose their medicare benefits if they are fired from a job.

8. **T   F**   Support workers provide most support services for home care.

MULTIPLE RESPONSE

From the list below, choose all of the correct answers.

9. The principles of medicare listed in the *Canada Health Act* are:
   A. Public administration
   B. Comprehensiveness
   C. Fairness to all
   D. Universality
   E. Transparency
   F. Portability
   G. Right to free speech
   H. Accessibility

Copyright © 2018 Elsevier Canada, a division of Reed Elsevier Canada, Ltd.

10. Professional services offered within home care services include:
    A. Nursing care
    B. Laundry services
    C. Physiotherapy
    D. Occupational therapy
    E. Speech therapy
    F. Massage therapy
    G. Cooking and housekeeping services
    H. Nutrition counselling
    I. Social work
    J. Respiratory therapy

11. *Health promotion* refers to strategies that:
    A. Assist a client with legal issues when needed
    B. Enhance or maintain a client's health
    C. Improve or sustain a client's independence

12. *Disease prevention* refers to strategies that:
    A. Prevent the occurrence of disease or injury
    B. Assist clients to improve their overall health
    C. Ensure acute-hospital funding
    D. Encourage a lifestyle of healthy eating and exercise
    E. Provide war veterans with psychological services if needed

13. Home care services today provide support to a large range of clients. These clients include:
    A. Women in labour
    B. Older adults
    C. Families with children
    D. Babies being treated in neonatal critical care units
    E. People with mental, physical, or developmental disabilities
    F. People with short-term medical conditions
    G. People with long-term medical conditions
    H. Inmates in a correctional facility
    I. Clients on telemetry (cardiac monitoring) in a coronary care unit
    J. People in the recovery stage, rehabilitative stage, or final stage of a life-ending disease

14. Examples of government policies that promote health and prevent illness are:
    A. Prenatal and parenting classes
    B. Immunization programs
    C. Same-sex marriage laws
    D. Driver's education programs
    E. Information campaigns (e.g., to reduce drinking during pregnancy, unsafe sex, and tobacco use)
    F. Age of majority legislation
    G. Efforts to improve housing, decrease poverty, monitor safe drinking water, and protect the environment

MULTIPLE CHOICE

Circle the correct answer.

15. As a support worker, you contribute to health promotion by:
    A. Providing medical care and services that can help prevent major health problems
    B. Providing end-of-life care to clients who are dying
    C. Smoking on your work breaks
    D. Placing soiled laundry immediately in the correct hamper instead of on the floor

16. In 2004, Tommy Douglas was voted "the Greatest Canadian." His main contribution to Saskatchewan as health minister was to initiate:
    A. A support worker program
    B. A free food program for the people in Saskatchewan
    C. 4 weeks of paid vacation time for everybody
    D. A medicare system

17. Private health insurance:
    A. Is available only to people who are in a low-income bracket
    B. Is illegal in Canada
    C. Must be paid for by either the client or the client's employer
    D. Is unnecessary because most people's provincial or territorial health insurance pays for all items

Copyright © 2018 Elsevier Canada, a division of Reed Elsevier Canada, Ltd.

18. Telehealth offers health care services by providing:
    A. Phone-in prescription services to pharmacies for clients
    B. Telephone advice from nurses to people who call in
    C. In-home supportive care
    D. The telephone numbers of local doctors who are accepting clients

19. An example of a health promotion strategy is a:
    A. "Stop smoking" advertising campaign
    B. Stroke recovery program for people who have had a stroke
    C. Campaign to hire more cancer doctors in a community
    D. Program that provides hearing aids for seniors

20. It is important to identify the key determinants of a community's health because they help predict which groups:
    A. Are most likely to develop health challenges
    B. Need to be taxed more, based on their lifestyle issues
    C. Are beyond help from the government
    D. Cannot change their unhealthy behaviours

MATCHING

Place the correct year next to the each statement below.

21. _____ No health insurance was available in Canada.   1961

22. _____ Saskatchewan introduced an insurance plan to cover hospital costs.   1947

23. _____ All provinces covered medical services provided outside hospitals.   1930

24. _____ All provinces covered inpatient hospital care.   1972

FILL IN THE BLANKS

For each of the following, mark P to indicate "professional service" or S to indicate "support service."

25. _____ Nursing care

26. _____ Physiotherapy

27. _____ Personal care

28. _____ Social work

29. _____ Assistance with activities of daily living

30. _____ Speech therapy

Copyright © 2018 Elsevier Canada, a division of Reed Elsevier Canada, Ltd.

Workplace Settings

TRUE OR FALSE

Circle T for true, or circle F for false.

1. **T   F**   Retirement residences are financed by the government.

2. **T   F**   Support workers are responsible for 80% of the total hours worked by all home care workers.

3. **T   F**   Some hospitals hire support workers.

4. **T   F**   In a community day program, the support worker works independently.

5. **T   F**   Working in a facility requires you to do many tasks in a limited period of time.

6. **T   F**   A lack of privacy can lead to loss of self-esteem.

7. **T   F**   Another term for *acute care* is *convalescent care.*

MULTIPLE RESPONSE

From the list below, choose all of the correct answers.

8. A persistent illness is an illness that:
   A. Is ongoing
   B. May worsen over time
   C. Usually has no cure
   D. Is always fatal

9. An acute illness is described as an illness:
   A. That appears suddenly
   B. That is recurrent and untreatable
   C. That lasts a short period of time
   D. That is mild and does not require medical treatment

10. Working in home care presents issues and challenges such as:
    A. Working on your own
    B. Taking direction from different professionals
    C. Undertaking difficult tasks such as shovelling snow
    D. Maintaining professional boundaries
    E. Providing for client safety
    F. Providing for personal safety
    G. Working with other team members

Copyright © 2018 Elsevier Canada, a division of Reed Elsevier Canada, Ltd.

11. What types of services do community day programs offer?
    A. Respite for family members
    B. Rehabilitation
    C. Counselling for people with mental health disorders
    D. Recreational activities
    E. Personal care services such as nail care

12. A residential facility provides care to people who:
    A. Are too young to live on their own
    B. Cannot care for themselves at home
    C. Can care for themselves independently but are too lonely to do so
    D. Require basic care but not acute medical care

13. The goals of long-term care are to:
    A. Provide care leading to a complete recovery or cure
    B. Maintain the clients' health and independence to the greatest extent possible
    C. Meet clients' physical, emotional, social, intellectual, and spiritual needs

14. Examples of a persistent (chronic) illness include:
    A. Bone fractures
    B. Diabetes
    C. Recent urinary tract infection
    D. Multiple sclerosis
    E. Appendicitis

15. Examples of acute illnesses include:
    A. Pneumonia
    B. Alzheimer's disease
    C. Influenza
    D. Kidney stone

MULTIPLE CHOICE

Circle the correct answer. Note: There is one correct answer for each.

16. Your client was admitted to a subacute-care facility. Another name for this is a(n):
    A. Convalescent care
    B. Hospital
    C. Outpatient facility
    D. Long-term care facility

17. Mrs. Jones receives community-based services. This means:
    A. She receives care in her community hospital
    B. She receives care after admission into a long-term care facility
    C. Her health care services are supplied outside of a facility
    D. She can receive care only in her home

18. A support worker can maintain professional boundaries with clients by:
    A. Refusing to drive a client to a medical appointment if asked
    B. Not discussing personal problems with clients
    C. Avoiding eye contact with clients or family members
    D. Giving out her home telephone number to clients

19. Often, employers will provide a newly hired worker with a written list of expected duties. Why should you ask for one if you have not received one? So you:
    A. Can find out which agency has the easiest set of duties
    B. Can negotiate which duty you want to eliminate
    C. Know what your co-workers should be doing
    D. Understand the full range of your duties

Copyright © 2018 Elsevier Canada, a division of Reed Elsevier Canada, Ltd.

20. Restoring a client to normal or near-normal function is the aim of which type of care?
    A. Respite care
    B. Rehabilitative care
    C. Assisted living
    D. Extended care

21. As a new graduate, you are able to demonstrate professional behaviour by:
    A. Seeking assistance before attempting a new procedure
    B. Attempting to do new treatments quickly and independently
    C. Being honest and telling the client that you have just learned this procedure
    D. Avoiding situations with clients that may be uncomfortable

22. In home care, support workers:
    A. Have a secondary role within home care.
    B. Are responsible for a wide range of home care services.
    C. Are hired on a part-time basis only.
    D. Do not have to take direction from others.

MATCHING

Match the type of service in the left column with the correct description in the right column.

23. Serves people and families living with progressive and life-threatening illness

24. Provides services to people who cannot care for themselves at home but do not need hospital care

25. Provides temporary care of a person who needs a high level of support

26. Provides services to people with immediate health issues

27. Provides rehabilitation for people recovering from surgery or injury

28. Provides therapies and education designed to restore or improve a person's independence

29. Provides services for people with mental health disorders

30. Provides care to people in their homes

A. Respite care
B. Home care
C. Palliative care
D. Acute care
E. Long-term care
F. Subacute care
G. Rehabilitation care
H. Mental health care

Copyright © 2018 Elsevier Canada, a division of Reed Elsevier Canada, Ltd.

Health, Wellness, Illness, and Disability

TRUE OR FALSE

Circle T for true, or circle F for false.

1. **T   F**   A formal group of people who help each other is called a *social support system.*

2. **T   F**   For some people, spiritual health is closely linked to religion.

3. **T   F**   Shamans are believed to use special powers to aid in the healing process.

4. **T   F**   Illness is the loss of physical or mental health.

5. **T   F**   Self-image is the individual's perception of himself or herself.

6. **T   F**   Choosing athletes for a team shows discrimination against those not chosen.

7. **T   F**   It is less stressful for your client if you make all the decisions on her behalf.

8. **T   F**   Changes in sexual function greatly affect some people.

MULTIPLE RESPONSE

From the list below, choose all of the correct answers.

9. *Health* is defined as a state of:
   A. Making a lot of money
   B. Complete physical, mental, and social well-being
   C. Well-being in all dimensions of one's life
   D. Not just the absence of disease or infirmity

10. What are the five dimensions of health?
    A. Physical health
    B. Emotional health
    C. Financial health
    D. Social health
    E. Cognitive health
    F. Religious health
    G. Spiritual health

Copyright © 2018 Elsevier Canada, a division of Reed Elsevier Canada, Ltd.

11. What factors contribute to physical health?
    A. Following a nutritious diet
    B. Having friends and companions
    C. Exercising regularly
    D. Living in a smoke-free environment
    E. Practising safe sex at all times
    F. Drinking alcohol moderately or not at all
    G. Having a good night's sleep
    H. Following safety practices
    I. Seeking medical attention when needed

12. How can you promote cognitive health for your clients?
    A. Encourage clients to participate in games and outings
    B. Take clients to religious services
    C. Encourage clients to read
    D. Help clients to do crossword puzzles or crafts
    E. Talk with clients about community and world events
    F. Encourage clients to toilet themselves

13. What are some of the factors affecting a person's experience of illness or disability?
    A. The nature of the illness or condition
    B. Age
    C. Level of physical fitness
    D. Amount of pain and discomfort
    E. The prognosis
    F. Emotional, social, cognitive, and spiritual health
    G. Personality and ability to cope with difficulties
    H. Culture
    I. The presence or absence of emotional, social, and financial support

14. Common reactions to illness or disability are:
    A. Joy and happiness
    B. Fear and anxiety
    C. Sadness and grief
    D. Depression
    E. Increased hunger
    F. Loss of bowel or bladder control
    G. Denial
    H. Anger

15. What are some of the changes and losses associated with illness and disability?
    A. Change in routine
    B. Increase in appetite
    C. Change in work life
    D. Change in family life
    E. Change in sexual function
    F. Loss of independence
    G. Loss of dignity
    H. Change in self-image
    I. Loss of intellect

MULTIPLE CHOICE

Circle the correct answer.

16. In the past, *health* was defined as:
    A. A fit, strong body
    B. The ability to function in society
    C. The absence of disease
    D. A belief in a higher being

17. A person's culture can influence health by:
    A. Causing poor working conditions
    B. Causing an inherited disease
    C. Influencing whom the person seeks health care from
    D. Making the person strong and resilient to illness

18. Determinants of health should be viewed in relation to each other and not just individually because:
    A. They are not very important by themselves
    B. They are poorly understood by themselves
    C. Canadians do not practise good health habits
    D. Each determinant can impact the other determinants

Copyright © 2018 Elsevier Canada, a division of Reed Elsevier Canada, Ltd.

19. Personal health practices and coping skills:
    A. Are not as important as genetics
    B. Are influenced by society and the people one is surrounded by
    C. Usually do not influence a person's ability to survive an illness
    D. Have never been linked to a healthy lifestyle

20. Holism:
    A. Is the consideration of a person's many dimensions
    B. Is not appropriate when a person has physical challenges
    C. Is a form of prejudice
    D. Is an outdated concept

MATCHING

Match the dimension of health with the correct definition.

21. _____ is achieved through an active, creative mind

22. _____ is achieved when the body is strong, fit, and free of disease

23. _____ is achieved through stable and satisfactory relationships

24. _____ results when people feel good about themselves

25. _____ is achieved through the belief in a purpose greater than the self

A. Physical health

B. Social health

C. Cognitive health

D. Spiritual health

E. Emotional health

Copyright © 2018 Elsevier Canada, a division of Reed Elsevier Canada, Ltd.

Interpersonal Communication

TRUE OR FALSE

Circle T for true, or circle F for false.

1. **T** **F** The same word can mean something different to two different people.

2. **T** **F** Touch is not a type of communication.

3. **T** **F** When paraphrasing, expand on the message and use more words to ensure you understand.

4. **T** **F** Nonverbal clues often reflect a client's true feelings.

5. **T** **F** Most older clients are not aware of your body language.

6. **T** **F** Closed questions can be answered with "yes" or "no."

7. **T** **F** Focusing is useful when a client rambles.

8. **T** **F** Short sentences are more clearly understood than long ones.

9. **T** **F** It is not important to be at eye level when communicating.

10. **T** **F** Using pet names such as "dear" can improve communication.

11. **T** **F** Assertive communication is the same as aggressive communication.

12. **T** **F** You can use open-ended questions to start a conversation.

13. **T** **F** Gestures, facial expressions, posture, body movements, touch, and appearance are ways of communicating without words.

14. **T** **F** When you hold a client's hand or touch the shoulder to convey caring or warmth, you are using verbal communication.

Copyright © 2018 Elsevier Canada, a division of Reed Elsevier Canada, Ltd.

15. **T   F**   A client who denies having pain but protects a body part by lying in a certain way is using body language to communicate.

16. **T   F**   When a support worker frowns or wrinkles the nose because the client has body odour, the support worker is sending a message through body language.

17. **T   F**   A support worker telling a client "Don't worry" or "Everything will be okay" may be a barrier to effective communication.

MULTIPLE RESPONSE

From the list below, choose all of the correct answers.

18. Body language includes which of the following?
    A. Appearance
    B. Facial expressions
    C. Posture
    D. Tone of voice
    E. Eye contact
    F. Gestures

19. To effectively communicate with words, you need to:
    A. Choose words carefully
    B. Pretend to understand
    C. Ask one question at a time
    D. Speak clearly, quickly, and distinctly
    E. Control your volume and tone of voice
    F. Be brief and concise
    G. Determine understanding
    H. Use simple, everyday language

20. Guidelines for active listening include:
    A. Making eye contact
    B. Facing the client
    C. Responding to the client
    D. Leaning toward the client

21. What are some of the barriers to good communication?
    A. Hearing impairment
    B. Vision impairment
    C. Nervous system disorders
    D. Too much privacy
    E. Cultural differences
    F. Loud noises
    G. Distractions

22. Nonverbal signs of anger include:
    A. Pacing
    B. Clenched fists
    C. Reddened face or neck
    D. Shouting
    E. Rapid movements

23. Clients feel safer and more secure during a procedure if you:
    A. Complete the procedure quickly
    B. Explain why and how the procedure is done
    C. Describe sensations or feelings they can expect
    D. Explain who will do it

24. Which of the following behaviours can create barriers to effective communication?
    A. Interrupting
    B. Giving advice
    C. Answering clients' questions
    D. Minimizing problems
    E. Using patronizing language
    F. Failing to listen

25. Which of the following are steps in the four-step teaching method used when teaching a client a task?
    A. Describe to the client the steps in the task
    B. Show the client how to do each task
    C. Have the client try each step
    D. Review what the client did wrong with each step

Copyright © 2018 Elsevier Canada, a division of Reed Elsevier Canada, Ltd.

26. Which of the following are some of the other guidelines you can use when you are teaching tasks to clients?
    A. Put the client at ease
    B. Start with small, easy steps
    C. Observe and listen
    D. Make sure you set the pace
    E. Allow for time to practise

27. Which of the following are the guidelines for dealing with an angry client?
    A. Ignore the client's feelings
    B. Treat the client with dignity and respect
    C. Tell the client what you are going to do and when
    D. Stay calm and professional
    E. Argue your point
    F. Listen and use silence
    G. Protect yourself from violent behaviours
    H. Report the client's behaviour to your supervisor

MULTIPLE CHOICE

Circle the correct answer.

28. *Interpersonal communication* is defined as:
    A. A verbal account of client care and observations
    B. A written account of care and observations
    C. The use of senses to collect information about a client
    D. The exchange of information between two people

29. When you communicate assertively, you appear:
    A. Cold or angry
    B. Hesitant and timid
    C. Intimidated
    D. Confident and calm

30. You are teaching Mr. Simpson how to change his ostomy bag. You would:
    A. Explain all the steps necessary before starting the demonstration
    B. Teach him the hardest part first
    C. Use positive statements for encouragement
    D. Set a time limit for him to complete the task

31. You are bathing Mrs. Fox when she suddenly starts to yell at you for not doing the bath correctly. Which of the following is an effective way to communicate with Mrs. Fox?
    A. Deny that you are doing it incorrectly
    B. Stay calm and professional
    C. Tell her you have been doing baths for many years and know what you are doing
    D. Stop the bath and leave the room

32. Asking closed questions:
    A. Invites a client to share thoughts or feelings
    B. Helps you to make sure you understand the client's message
    C. Focuses on obtaining specific information
    D. Helps you to find out about the client's needs

Copyright © 2018 Elsevier Canada, a division of Reed Elsevier Canada, Ltd.

MATCHING

Match the term with the definition.

33. _____ Giving an acceptable reason or excuse for one's behaviour or actions

34. _____ Transferring one's behaviour or emotions from one person, place, or thing to another

35. _____ Keeping unpleasant or painful thoughts or experiences from the conscious mind

36. _____ Directing emotions toward another person or thing that seems safe rather than toward the person or thing that is the source of the emotions

37. _____ Refusing to face or accept something that is unpleasant

38. _____ Acting in a way that is opposite to what one truly feels

39. _____ Retreating or moving back to an earlier time or condition

A. Denial

B. Displacement

C. Projection

D. Regression

E. Rationalization

F. Repression

G. Reaction formation

Match the description with the correct term.

40. _____ Restating someone's message in your own words

41. _____ Communicating positively and directly without offending others

42. _____ Questions that invite a client to share thoughts

43. _____ Paying close attention to a client's verbal and nonverbal communication

44. _____ Questions that focus on specific information

45. _____ Being attentive to a client's feelings

46. _____ Messages sent without words

47. _____ Limiting the conversation to a certain topic

48. _____ Gestures that send messages to others

49. _____ Spoken words

50. _____ Exchange of information between two people

A. Open-ended questions

B. Nonverbal communication

C. Paraphrasing

D. Verbal communication

E. Closed questions

F. Interpersonal communication

G. Empathetic listening

H. Body language

I. Active listening

J. Focusing

K. Assertiveness

Copyright © 2018 Elsevier Canada, a division of Reed Elsevier Canada, Ltd.

FILL IN THE BLANKS

51. The communication process involves the following steps:

   a. _____

   b. _____

   c. _____

   d. _____

52. You can use open-ended questions to

   a. _____

   b. _____

Copyright © 2018 Elsevier Canada, a division of Reed Elsevier Canada, Ltd.

Working With Others: Teamwork, Supervision, and Delegation

TRUE OR FALSE

Circle T for true, or circle F for false.

1. **T   F**   You can be delegated an authorized act only if it is allowed within your job description and your employer's policy.

2. **T   F**   Registered practical nurses are not allowed to supervise support workers.

3. **T   F**   It is okay to discuss work problems with your client as long as you do not use proper names.

4. **T   F**   When you agree to perform a task, you are responsible for your own actions.

5. **T   F**   You may refuse a delegated task if you do not want to do the task.

6. **T   F**   Delegating is the same as supervising.

7. **T   F**   Support workers are allowed to perform procedures below the skin surface.

MULTIPLE RESPONSE

From the list below, choose all of the correct answers.

8. Which of the following are benefits of working on a team?
   A. Opportunities for collaboration
   B. Opportunities for communication
   C. Working with people who have a wide range of abilities, skills, and perspectives
   D. Better decision making and problem solving
   E. Dealing with conflict

9. Which of the following are usually members of the health care team in a long-term care facility?
   A. Physician
   B. Nurse
   C. Dietitian
   D. Client
   E. Personal support worker
   F. Case manager
   G. Volunteer

10. When the nurse delegates a task to you in a facility, he or she is required to do which of the following?
    A. Monitor you over time to ensure you remain able to perform the task correctly and safely
    B. Assess your base of knowledge
    C. Teach you the task
    D. Make sure it is within your scope of practice
    E. Assess your performance

11. Which of the following concerns will affect delegation decisions?
    A. What is the client's condition?
    B. What are the risks involved?
    C. Can the support worker be adequately supervised?
    D. Will the support worker be required to perform the task frequently?
    E. Does the support worker want to perform the task?
    F. What tasks are included in the support worker's job description?

12. Teams in home care usually include which of the following?
    A. Family members
    B. Client
    C. Personal support worker
    D. Nurse
    E. Neighbours
    F. Case manager
    G. Social worker
    H. Physician

MULTIPLE CHOICE

Circle the correct answer.

13. When the nurse delegates a task to a support worker, who is accountable for the delegated task?
    A. The nurse
    B. The support worker
    C. The case manager
    D. The doctor

14. Which of the following is NOT one of the five rights?
    A. Right directions and communication
    B. Right supervision
    C. Right equipment
    D. Right circumstances

15. Which of the following is NOT an appropriate reason for a support worker to refuse a task? He or she:
    A. Is not trained to perform the task safely
    B. Does not know the client or resident
    C. Knows the task will require staying at work late
    D. Does not like the nurse who asked him or her to perform the task

16. Which of the following activities would be acceptable while you are at work?
    A. Making a copy of your paycheque on the photocopier
    B. Planning to eat lunch with your sister
    C. Leaving a half-hour early for a doctor's appointment
    D. None of the above

17. What are some of the challenges to working on a team?
    A. Making better decisions
    B. Having opportunities for communication
    C. Working with people who have a wide array of abilities
    D. Recognizing role boundaries

Copyright © 2018 Elsevier Canada, a division of Reed Elsevier Canada, Ltd.

18. A controlled act is a task that:
    A. Must be performed only by those
        authorized to perform it.
    B. All support workers can do on home
        care clients.
    C. All health care team members can
        perform.
    D. Must be authorized to be performed on
        a daily basis.

MATCHING

Match the terms with the correct definition.

19. _____ To work together toward a common goal

20. _____ The nurse on duty for that shift

21. _____ Person who assesses the client's needs in the
            community

22. _____ Transfer of function

23. _____ A function you perform for the client

24. _____ The legal right

A. Delegation

B. Task

C. Case manager

D. Collaborate

E. Charge nurse

F. Authority

Match the correct Right of Delegation with the question the support worker should ask himself or herself before performing an assigned task.

25. _____ Do I have concerns about performing the task?

26. _____ Do I feel competent in performing the task?

27. _____ Is a nurse available if the client's condition changes
            or if problems occur?

28. _____ Was I trained to do the task?

29. _____ Did I review the task with a nurse?

A. Right task

B. Right circumstances

C. Right person

D. Right directions and communication

E. Right supervision and evaluation

Copyright © 2018 Elsevier Canada, a division of Reed Elsevier Canada, Ltd.

Managing Stress, Time, and Problems

TRUE OR FALSE

Circle T for true, or circle F for false.

1.   **T**   **F**   Stressors over a short period of time can cause a persistent illness.

2.   **T**   **F**   You should set weekly goals for yourself.

3.   **T**   **F**   Getting a promotion can cause stress.

4.   **T**   **F**   A child usually shows different signs of stress from those of an adult.

5.   **T**   **F**   Time management is essential to reducing stress.

6.   **T**   **F**   There is no point in planning your work a day ahead because things change when you get to work.

7.   **T**   **F**   You don't need to report a conflict with a client if it is resolved.

8.   **T**   **F**   In a home care setting, you must plan your time so you can be on time for the next client.

9.   **T**   **F**   Older adults are less able to cope with stress than younger adults.

10.   **T**   **F**   All stress is bad for your well-being.

MULTIPLE RESPONSE

From the list below, choose all of the correct answers.

11.   Which of the following strategies can help you manage stress in your life?
A.   Think positively.
B.   Develop self-awareness.
C.   Ask for help and support.
D.   Be aggressive.
E.   Practise calming exercises.

12.   Which of the following can help you save time and stay organized?
A.   Identify priorities.
B.   Set goals.
C.   Multi-task.
D.   Make daily plans.
E.   Make a weekly plan.

Copyright © 2018 Elsevier Canada, a division of Reed Elsevier Canada, Ltd.

13. Which of the following strategies can you use to manage conflict at work?
    A. Identify and solve problems before they become major issues.
    B. Explain the situation to a co-worker and ask for advice.
    C. Arrange a private meeting with the person with whom you have a conflict.
    D. Explain the problem to the person, focusing on the facts, not on the person.
    E. Listen to the other person's response without interrupting.

14. Which of the following can be physical signs of stress?
    A. Rapid pulse
    B. Rapid respirations
    C. Decreased blood pressure
    D. Slow speech
    E. Difficulty swallowing
    F. Difficulty sleeping

15. Emotional and behavioural signs of stress can include which of the following?
    A. Anxiety
    B. Depression
    C. Anger
    D. Increased self-esteem
    E. Poor concentration
    F. Drinking

16. Which of the following represent the acronym *SMART* when referring to goals?
    A. Specific
    B. Simple
    C. Measurable
    D. Manageable
    E. Achievable
    F. Reliable
    G. Realistic
    H. Timely
    I. Team

MULTIPLE CHOICE

Circle the correct answer.

17. Which of the following defines *anxiety*?
    A. An unconscious reaction that blocks unpleasant feelings
    B. A state of exhaustion
    C. An event that causes stress
    D. A vague, uneasy feeling

18. Which of the following defines *projection*?
    A. Assigning one's feelings to someone or something else
    B. Acting in a way that is opposite to what you feel
    C. Reverting or moving back to earlier behaviours
    D. Changing an emotion into a physical reaction

19. Which of the following is a physical sign of stress?
    A. Forgetfulness
    B. Fear
    C. Sweaty palms
    D. Anger

20. Which strategy will help you manage stress?
    A. Sleeping more
    B. Developing self-awareness
    C. Trying to manage everything yourself
    D. None of the above

21. You may encounter conflict with the client's family members because:
    A. They are just being difficult
    B. They want to be in control
    C. They do not understand the nursing care plan
    D. They do not like you

Copyright © 2018 Elsevier Canada, a division of Reed Elsevier Canada, Ltd.

MATCHING

Match the term with the definition.

22. _____ A vague, uneasy feeling, often including a sense of impending danger or harm

23. _____ The emotional, behavioural, or physical response to an event or situation

24. _____ Symptom state of physical, emotional, and mental exhaustion

25. _____ Ongoing stress that can lead to burnout

26. _____ To acknowledge, recognize, or confirm the person's feelings.

27. _____ A type of stressor that is healthy and gives one the feeling of fulfilment

28. _____ A clash between opposing interests and ideas

29. _____ An event or situation that causes stress

A. Burnout

B. Eustress

C. Validate

D. Stress

E. Stressor

F. Anxiety

G. Chronic stress

H. Conflict

FILL IN THE BLANKS

30. Problem solving is a process. Describe this process.

_____

_____

_____

_____

_____

31. What are some common stressors you may face?

a. _____

b. _____

c. _____

d. _____

e. _____

Copyright © 2018 Elsevier Canada, a division of Reed Elsevier Canada, Ltd.

32. When you realize you have a problem at work, when should you consult your supervisor?

    a. _____

    b. _____

    c. _____

    d. _____

    e. _____

33. What steps should be taken to resolve a conflict between two people?

    a. _____

    b. _____

    c. _____

    d. _____

    e. _____

    f. _____

    g. _____

    h. _____

    i. _____

    j. _____

    k. _____

Copyright © 2018 Elsevier Canada, a division of Reed Elsevier Canada, Ltd.

Ethics

TRUE OR FALSE

Circle T for true, or circle F for false.

1. T   F   Support workers have a formal code of ethics.

2. T   F   Clients have the right to refuse a treatment they do not want.

3. T   F   You can uphold the principle of justice by being concerned about all clients.

4. T   F   It is okay to talk about a client in the locker room.

5. T   F   There is nothing wrong with accepting a dinner invitation from a member of a client's family.

6. T   F   A support worker is free to discuss a client's progress or treatment with a close family member.

7. T   F   You should not take sides with a client against a family member.

8. T   F   Becoming personally involved with clients or their family members may prevent you from providing nonjudgemental care.

MULTIPLE RESPONSE

From the list below, choose all of the correct answers.

9. *Ethics* refers to:
   A.   Laws that govern our community
   B.   Beliefs that determine what is good or bad
   C.   Guidelines that help us to decide what is right or wrong
   D.   Moral principles or values that guide our choices

10. Which points should be included in a sample code of ethics for support workers?
    A.   Provide high-quality personal care and support services
    B.   Provide compassionate care to paying clients only
    C.   Value the dignity of all clients
    D.   Respect clients' choices about how they receive or participate in their care
    E.   Respect clients' rights to privacy and confidentiality
    F.   Do not misuse the support worker's position of trust
    G.   Be reliable most of the time
    H.   Promote and maintain clients' safety

Copyright © 2018 Elsevier Canada, a division of Reed Elsevier Canada, Ltd.

11. The four basic principles of health care ethics are:
    A. Autonomy
    B. Honesty
    C. Justice
    D. Beneficence
    E. Maleficence
    F. Nonmaleficence

12. Which of the following points will *correctly* assist you to decide on a course of action when faced with an ethical dilemma involving a client?
    A. Consider the five principles of health care ethics
    B. Collect as much information about the situation as possible
    C. Consider a few of your available options
    D. Determine if the action provides you with a short-term or long-term benefit
    E. Consider if the action will treat the client justly and fairly
    F. Decide if the action can cause harm or increase the risk of harm to the client
    G. Consider the client's wishes and preferences before deciding

MULTIPLE CHOICE

Circle the correct answer.

13. Ethics is:
    A. Concerned with what is right and wrong behaviour
    B. About making bad judgements before knowing the facts
    C. Deciding whether a situation is right or wrong based on your own life experiences
    D. A law telling you what you can and cannot do

14. You ask Ms. Burton if she is ready to get dressed. She says, "I would like to wait until after breakfast." She is exercising her right to:
    A. Privacy
    B. Freedom from abuse, mistreatment, and neglect
    C. Personal choice
    D. Be free from restraint

15. Ms. Burton will not consent to a physical examination. She is exercising her right to:
    A. Personal choice
    B. Privacy
    C. Quality of life
    D. Refuse treatment

16. Ms. Burton continues to refuse to take a shower. Which is true?
    A. The staff can force Ms. Burton to shower.
    B. Ms. Burton's family should force her to shower.
    C. The staff needs to first find out why she refuses to shower.
    D. The staff should immediately report Ms. Burton's refusal to the supervisor.

17. *Work ethics* refers to:
    A. Trusting others with information
    B. Being polite and considerate
    C. Behaviour in the workplace
    D. Right and wrong conduct

18. An example of just treatment includes:
    A. Treating everybody with fairness
    B. Talking about others in the cafeteria
    C. Avoiding a client whose lifestyle you do not approve of
    D. Lying about someone to avoid embarrassment

Copyright © 2018 Elsevier Canada, a division of Reed Elsevier Canada, Ltd.

MATCHING

Match each definition with the correct term.

19. Seeking to do no harm   A. Autonomy

20. Doing or promoting good   B. Justice

21. Abuse   C. Beneficence

22. All people should be treated in a fair manner   D. Intentional harm

23. Accidental injury or negligence   E. Nonmaleficence

24. Having free choice   F. Unintentional harm

FILL IN THE BLANKS

25. What do you do if your client's choice may put him or her at risk for injury?

_____

_____

Copyright © 2018 Elsevier Canada, a division of Reed Elsevier Canada, Ltd.

Legislation: The Client's Rights and Your Rights

TRUE OR FALSE

Circle T for true, or circle F for false.

1. T   F   Employment standards and legislation protect you from harassment.

2. T   F   Libel is making false statements in print.

3. T   F   The unnecessary use of restraints is false imprisonment.

4. T   F   Civil laws deal with relationships between people.

5. T   F   A physician can ask you to obtain consent from a client.

6. T   F   You may refuse to do something beyond your scope of practice.

7. T   F   A common act of courtesy is one way to respect a client's dignity.

8. T   F   It is okay to open a client's mail in case it contains upsetting news.

9. T   F   Respecting a client's dignity can encourage independence.

10. T   F   It is important to tell the nurse when you leave the unit for meals and breaks and when you return to the unit.

11. T   F   Human rights legislation protects against harassment.

Copyright © 2018 Elsevier Canada, a division of Reed Elsevier Canada, Ltd.

MULTIPLE RESPONSE

From the list below, choose all of the correct answers.

12. Basic human rights in Canada include:
    A. The right to equality before and under the law, without discrimination based on race, ethnic origin, colour, religion, sex, age, or disability
    B. Freedom of action
    C. Freedom of thought, belief, opinion, and expression
    D. Freedom of peaceful assembly and association
    E. The right to drive
    F. The right to vote
    G. The right to enter, remain in, and leave Canada
    H. The right for illegal immigrants to stay in Canada
    I. The right to life, liberty, and security of the person
    J. Freedom of conscience and religion

13. Most long-term care facilities have policies that recognize that residents have the following rights:
    A. To be treated with dignity and respect
    B. To live in a safe and clean environment
    C. To be properly sheltered, clothed, groomed, and cared for
    D. To keep and display personal possessions, pictures, and furnishings in their rooms
    E. To have family present 24 hours a day if the person is dying
    F. To have hairdressing and barber services provided free of charge
    G. To be free from abuse
    H. To discuss problems or suggest changes to any aspect of the services provided to them
    I. To privacy and confidentiality
    J. To give or withhold informed consent
    K. To autonomy (the right to make decisions)

14. How can you show respect to your clients?
    A. Be courteous
    B. Respect the person's belongings and property
    C. Avoid eye contact
    D. Try to do as much as you can for the client
    E. Assist with personal care and grooming whenever—and only if—necessary
    F. Be patient
    G. Listen attentively
    H. Address an adult by title and last name, unless the person tells you to do otherwise
    I. Never scold, laugh at, or embarrass the person

15. Informed consent for a treatment should include knowledge about:
    A. Potential risks and side effects of the treatment
    B. The reason for the treatment or service
    C. How the treatment will be done
    D. Who will be doing the treatment
    E. The expected outcomes
    F. What will be done during the treatment
    G. Other treatment options
    H. The health care worker's opinions of the treatment
    I. The likely consequences of not having the treatment

MULTIPLE CHOICE

Circle the correct answer.

16. If a client has different values or standards from yours, you should:
    A. Respect the client as an individual
    B. Refuse to care for the client
    C. Firmly tell the client what your values are
    D. Discuss the client's beliefs with others at work or at home

Copyright © 2018 Elsevier Canada, a division of Reed Elsevier Canada, Ltd.

17. If you are asked to obtain a client's signature on an informed consent form, you should:
    A. Make sure the client is mentally competent
    B. Refuse because this is not a support worker's responsibility
    C. Ask a family member to witness the signature
    D. Call the doctor to witness the signature

18. If a client refuses treatment, what action should be taken by the health care facility?
    A. Give the treatment as ordered
    B. Honour the request and discontinue the treatment
    C. Find out what the client is refusing and why
    D. Tell the family that the client must be removed from the facility

19. A client tells you he is upset because he believes his treatment was done incorrectly yesterday. Your action is based on which of the following?
    A. He has a right to voice his concerns and to have the facility try to correct the matter
    B. You know the treatment was done correctly
    C. He complains constantly, so everyone ignores his concerns and questions
    D. He is confused and forgets what was done yesterday

20. What rights do clients have?
    A. They may discuss concerns and offer ideas
    B. They may take part in social, cultural, religious, and community activities
    C. They may receive support and reassurance from family members and friends
    D. All of the above

21. What action by the support worker protects the client's right to personal possessions?
    A. Throwing away old cards, letters, and magazines to tidy the unit
    B. Rearranging personal items so they are more decorative
    C. Getting the client's permission to look for an item in the closet
    D. Taking a piece of candy from the client's candy dish when he or she is not present

22. An advance directive is:
    A. The care plan
    B. An order not to resuscitate the client
    C. A legal document stating the client's wishes about future health care, treatment, and personal care
    D. A document stating the client's wishes about his or her personal belongings

23. A legal right is something that a person:
    A. Must earn by getting a job
    B. Must be a certain age to get
    C. Is entitled to in Canada
    D. Can get by applying for it from the government

24. When a client complains to you about the home care agency's policies, you should:
    A. Defend the agency and the policy
    B. Check the client's mental status on the care plan
    C. Inform your supervisor of the complaint
    D. Act interested and record it in your notepad

Copyright © 2018 Elsevier Canada, a division of Reed Elsevier Canada, Ltd.

25. A living will addresses the client's wishes about:
    A. Preferences about the care used to sustain the client's life
    B. Care and guardianship of the client's young children
    C. Having a tree planted in the client's name
    D. Who will receive the client's assets and property once the client has died

26. Who is responsible for job safety in a long-term care facility?
    A. The clients
    B. The maintenance staff who repair broken equipment
    C. Both employers and employees
    D. The provincial minister of health

27. An *act* is another term for:
    A. Standard
    B. Policy
    C. Law
    D. Licence

MATCHING

From the list provided, choose the word that best fills in the blank in each statement.

28. Making a false written statement that hurts the reputation of another is called _____.

29. Discussing a client's treatment with your best friend invades the client's _____.

30. In order to protect the client's right to privacy, the client's body must not be needlessly _____.

31. Consent is needed for _____ to observe the client's care.

32. The client has the right to _____ and _____ mail without interference.

33. Information about the client's _____, _____, and condition is kept confidential.

34. An individual has failed to act in a reasonable and careful manner and caused harm to the person or the person's property. This is a tort known as _____.

35. A support worker opens a client's mail and reads it. This is a tort known as _____.

A. Care; treatment

B. Privacy

C. Libel

D. Negligence

E. Invasion of privacy

F. Others

G. Send; receive

H. Exposed (or uncovered)

Copyright © 2018 Elsevier Canada, a division of Reed Elsevier Canada, Ltd.

From the list provided, choose the word that best fills in the blank in each statement.

36. After her morning care is completed, a client wants to do activities. The support worker does not allow the client to go. This is a tort known as _____.

37. A living will addresses the client's wishes about his _____ when he is at a point when he cannot speak for himself.

38. While cleaning a client's dentures, the support worker drops and breaks them. This is a tort known as _____.

39. Instead of allowing the client a choice, the support worker tells the client that she will get a shower whether or not she wants one. This is a tort known as _____.

40. An individual makes defamatory statements about another person. This is a tort known as _____.

41. A support worker talks to employees from other departments about a client. This is a tort known as _____.

42. Your best protection against charges of negligence is _____ every procedure.

43. The client is allowed to visit family and friends in _____.

A. Slander

B. Assault

C. Documenting (or recording)

D. Private

E. Negligence

F. False imprisonment

G. Care

H. Invasion of privacy

Copyright © 2018 Elsevier Canada, a division of Reed Elsevier Canada, Ltd.

From the list provided, choose the word that best fills in the blank in each statement.

44. A client pressed the call bell 20 minutes ago. When no one responds, he tries to go to the bathroom alone, slips and falls, and breaks a hip. This is a tort known as _____.

45. An individual has injured the name and reputation of a person by making false statements to a third person. This is a tort known as _____.

46. An individual attempts or threatens to touch another person's body without the person's consent. This is a tort known as _____.

47. An individual touches another person's body without the person's consent. This is a tort known as _____.

48. An individual exposes the private affairs of another person to a third person. This is a tort known as _____.

49. An individual restrains or restricts another person's freedom of movement without a physician's order. This is a tort known as _____.

50. A worker causing harm to a person deliberately is called an _____ act.

51. A will addresses the client's wishes about personal _____.

A. Invasion of privacy

B. Intentional

C. Negligence

D. False imprisonment

E. Slander

F. Assault

G. Battery

H. Property

Match the words and definitions.

52. _____ What you should or should not do

53. _____ Having free choice

54. _____ Legally responsible

55. _____ Wrongful act committed against a person or a person's property

56. _____ A body of laws

57. _____ Failing to act in a competent manner

58. _____ Touching a person's body without consent

59. _____ Injuring the reputation of a person by making false statements

60. _____ Specific law

61. _____ Something to which a person is justly entitled

A. Right

B. Legislation

C. Liable

D. Negligence

E. Ethics

F. Act

G. Autonomy

H. Battery

I. Defamation

J. Tort

Copyright © 2018 Elsevier Canada, a division of Reed Elsevier Canada, Ltd.

FILL IN THE BLANKS

62. Informed consent is based on _____ and _____.

63. If a patient complains of chest pain and you do not report this to your supervisor, this is a _____ _____ act.

64. Discussing a person's treatment with your best friend invades the person's _____ _____.

65. List the ways you can protect a client's right to privacy.

    a. _____

    b. _____

    c. _____

    d. _____

    e. _____

    f. _____

    g. _____

    h. _____

66. What can cause negligence?

    a. _____

    b. _____

    c. _____

67. What are some of the laws that protect workers?

    a. _____

    b. _____

    c. _____

    d. _____

    e. _____

    f. _____

68. Who is responsible for job safety?

    _____

69. A will addresses the client's wishes about _____, whereas a living will addresses the client's wishes about _____.

Copyright © 2018 Elsevier Canada, a division of Reed Elsevier Canada, Ltd.

Caring About Culture and Diversity

TRUE OR FALSE

Circle T for true, or circle F for false.

1. T F People of all cultures are comfortable with physical touch.

2. T F In Western cultures, personal space is about 120 cm (4 feet).

3. T F Silence can be a sign of respect in some cultures.

4. T F Some children rebel against the culture of their parents.

5. T F You should never try to convert your clients to your own belief system.

6. T F All folk remedies are harmless.

7. T F Discrimination leads to prejudice.

8. T F In some cultures, men do not shake women's hands.

9. T F Culture is influenced by a large number of factors.

10. T F Asking about your client's beliefs and values will help him or her feel valued and respected.

MULTIPLE RESPONSE

From the list below, choose all of the correct answers.

11. Culture affects a person's beliefs and behaviour in the areas of:
    A. Communication
    B. Receiving wages and earnings
    C. Family and social organization
    D. Religion and worship
    E. Health care practices and reactions to illness
    F. Body shape and intelligence

12. Qualities that support workers should possess include:
    A. Being respectful to all others
    B. Good listening skills
    C. Willingness to change people
    D. Understanding and accepting of other people's differences
    E. Awareness of body language

Copyright © 2018 Elsevier Canada, a division of Reed Elsevier Canada, Ltd.

13. Many facial expressions that convey emotions are universal; some of these expressions are to convey:
    A. Anger
    B. Pain
    C. Surprise
    D. Embarrassment
    E. Happiness

14. An extended family may include:
    A. Parents
    B. Grandparents
    C. Neighbours
    D. Friends
    E. Children
    F. Aunts
    G. Cousins

15. Religions may promote beliefs and practices related to:
    A. Daily living habits
    B. Behaviours
    C. Relationships with others
    D. Diet
    E. Healing
    F. Days of worship
    G. Birth and birth control
    H. Medicine
    I. Death

16. To be accepting and understanding of others, you need to understand:
    A. Everything about other cultures
    B. How your culture has influenced you
    C. How culture influences clients' behaviours and attitudes
    D. That all people are the same
    E. That each client is unique, and individuals may not follow every belief and practice of their culture or religion

17. When you communicate with people who don't speak your language, you should:
    A. Convey comfort by the tone of your voice and with your body language
    B. Speak loudly or shout your message
    C. Speak slowly and distinctly
    D. Keep messages short and simple
    E. Be alert for words the client seems to understand
    F. Use gestures and pictures
    G. Repeat the message, using the same words, so they understand you
    H. Use slang terms because these are usually understood
    I. Be certain the client understands what is going to happen and consents to a procedure before you begin it
    J. Learn a few useful phrases in the client's language

18. The acronym LGBTQ refers to a community of people who identify themselves as:
    A. Questioning their sexuality
    B. Transgender
    C. Transvestite
    D. Bisexual
    E. Straight
    F. Gay
    G. Lesbian
    H. Blended

MULTIPLE CHOICE

Circle the correct answer.

19. People of Asian background may conceal negative emotions with a:
    A. Laugh
    B. Smile
    C. Frown
    D. Stare

Copyright © 2018 Elsevier Canada, a division of Reed Elsevier Canada, Ltd.

20. Sam and Chris are a couple who share parenting responsibilities for two children. Sam is the parent of one of the children, but both Sam and Chris are the legal parents of the other child. This is an example of a _____ family.
    A. Blended
    B. Nuclear
    C. Single-parent
    D. Separated

21. Culture is considered to be more than just a person's ethnicity because:
    A. It can refer to characteristics learned by living in any group (e.g., a group of college students)
    B. Most Canadians do not have an ethnic background
    C. Ethnicity has nothing to do with culture
    D. There is no such thing as ethnicity

22. Jim is a homosexual man who was recently beaten up after leaving a gay bar with a friend. This is an example of:
    A. Racism
    B. Ageism
    C. Homophobia
    D. Sexism

23. Tony's parents came to Canada from Italy when Tony was 3 years old. He is expected to marry someone who is also of Italian descent. However, Tony is seriously dating someone from an Asian background. This situation is an example of:
    A. Cultural stereotyping
    B. Cultural conflict
    C. Ethnic cleansing
    D. Ethnic identity

24. A nuclear family consists of a:
    A. Mother, father, and children
    B. Mother, father, children, and grandparents
    C. Mother and children
    D. Father, father, and children

25. Gayle has refused to take her prescribed blood pressure medication because of her religious faith. However, her family would like you to "sneak" her pills into her by grinding them and adding them to her food. Your best response to her family would be:
    A. "If you want me to do this, it'll cost you money!"
    B. "Are you kidding? I could get fired for this!"
    C. "It would be wrong for me to go against a client's wishes."
    D. "Why don't you do it while I leave the room?"

26. Mrs. Jing, who is a Buddhist, would like to pray and has asked if you could pray with her. You practise a different faith. What should you say to her request?
    A. "I'm not a member of that religion. Let me find someone who is."
    B. "No way. I don't believe in any of that."
    C. "I am not allowed to pray with clients."
    D. "I will support you while you pray as long as I am able."

27. Sue would like to get a job as a construction worker. She was denied because she might get pregnant and require a maternity leave. This is an example of:
    A. Cultural conflict
    B. Sexism
    C. Racism
    D. Ethnic identity

28. Mr. Jones has asked for a male support worker because according to his religion, it is improper to be touched by a female other than his wife. There are no male support workers working that day. How should you handle this situation?
    A. Speak to your supervisor about the situation immediately
    B. Tell Mr. Jones that you are the only one available and that he should be happy to get any care at all
    C. Care for him but wear gloves to avoid skin-to-skin contact
    D. Tell him to do his own care

Copyright © 2018 Elsevier Canada, a division of Reed Elsevier Canada, Ltd.

MATCHING

Match the terms and definitions.

29. _____ Characteristics of a group of people

30. _____ An overly simple or exaggerated impression of a person

31. _____ The unfair treatment of people based on their group membership

32. _____ The area immediately around one's body

33. _____ Groups of people who share similar physical features

34. _____ Groups of people who share a common history

35. _____ An attitude that judges a person based on his or her membership in a group

A. Race

B. Prejudice

C. Ethnic group

D. Culture

E. Personal space

F. Stereotype

G. Discrimination

FILL IN THE BLANKS

36. Culture affects a person's beliefs and behaviour toward

   a. _____

   b. _____

   c. _____

   d. _____

37. Nonverbal cues can include

   a. _____

   b. _____

   c. _____

   d. _____

38. How can cultural conflict affect an older person? _____

   _____

39. Adopting the traditions of the larger society is called _____.

Copyright © 2018 Elsevier Canada, a division of Reed Elsevier Canada, Ltd.

Working With Clients and Their Families

TRUE OR FALSE

Circle T for true, or circle F for false.

1. **T** **F** Sympathy is the same as empathy.

2. **T** **F** Independence is the state of not depending on others for control.

3. **T** **F** When abused children become adults, they may abuse their own children.

4. **T** **F** You can be both a friend and a professional helper to your client.

5. **T** **F** Respect is showing acceptance and regard for another person.

MULTIPLE RESPONSE

From the list below, choose all of the correct answers.

6. When a procedure is performed, which of the following actions would demonstrate that the support worker is meeting the client's safety needs?
   A. Explains why the procedure needs to be done
   B. Describes how the resident in the next room handled the procedure
   C. Explains who will do the procedure
   D. Explains how the procedure will be performed
   E. Describes what sensations or feelings to expect

Copyright © 2018 Elsevier Canada, a division of Reed Elsevier Canada, Ltd.

7. Which of the following represent different types of families you may work with?
   A. A married couple with or without children
   B. An unmarried couple living together, with or without children
   C. A widowed grandparent raising grandchildren
   D. A divorced parent living with a partner
   E. Two women or two men living together in a same-sex relationship
   F. Older parents, adult children, and grandchildren living together

8. Which of the following are factors that can influence psychosocial health?
   A. Personality
   B. Family background
   C. Environment
   D. Disease
   E. Life circumstances

9. Which of the following are elements of a professional helping relationship?
   A. There is a defined role within the relationship
   B. People involved may not choose the relationship
   C. The helper is judgemental
   D. One person takes responsibility for helping the other
   E. Both people in the relationship seek to have their needs fulfilled

MULTIPLE CHOICE

Circle the correct answer.

10. Feeling compassion for or understanding the difficulties of another person is the definition for:
    A. Compassion
    B. Respect
    C. Empathy
    D. Sympathy

11. Being competent means you must
    A. Seek and participate in lifelong learning
    B. Be flexible when making decisions.
    C. Take direction well from your supervisor
    D. Act professional at all times

12. Which is an indicator of a professional relationship versus a friendship?
    A. The relationship is not goal-directed
    B. The helper is nonjudgemental
    C. Both people may be judgemental
    D. Behaviours are based on personal roles

13. Empathy involves:
    A. Recognizing and understanding another person's emotions
    B. The desire and actions to reduce problems
    C. Offering advice and solutions
    D. Desiring to change the person's behaviour

14. Dependence is the state of:
    A. Relying on others for support
    B. Relying on each other for support
    C. Not depending on others
    D. None of the above

Copyright © 2018 Elsevier Canada, a division of Reed Elsevier Canada, Ltd.

MATCHING

Match the description below to its correct term.

15. _____ Being unable to manage without help

16. _____ Expressions of anger or irritation

17. _____ Not having to rely on others for control

18. _____ The state of relying on one another

19. _____ The ability to do a job well

20. _____ Acceptance and regard for another person

21. _____ Thinking well of oneself

22. _____ Understanding one's own feelings and moods

A. Respect

B. Self-awareness

C. Self-esteem

D. Independence

E. Conflict

F. Interdependence

G. Dependence

H. Competence

FILL IN THE BLANKS

23. How can you show your client respect?

a. _____

b. _____

c. _____

d. _____

24. Describe the difference between a professional helping relationship and a friendship.

_____

Copyright © 2018 Elsevier Canada, a division of Reed Elsevier Canada, Ltd.

Promoting Client Well-Being, Comfort, and Sleep

TRUE OR FALSE

Circle T for true, or circle F for false.

1. **T** **F** Personal items in a client's space are arranged as the individual prefers.

2. **T** **F** The support worker may throw away any items in the client's space that are in the way.

3. **T** **F** Make sure the client can reach the telephone, television, and light controls.

4. **T** **F** Moving furniture or belongings may be a safety hazard for a client with poor vision.

5. **T** **F** *Distraction* involves creating an image in the mind.

6. **T** **F** Older clients are at greater risk for undetected disease or injury because they have decreased pain sensations.

7. **T** **F** Crying, fussing, and changes in behaviour are normal in infants and young children.

8. **T** **F** Clients from birth to 1 year and clients 65 years and over will probably need lower room temperatures.

MULTIPLE RESPONSE

From the list below, choose all of the correct answers.

9. Which of the following are factors that affect pain?
   A. Past experience
   B. Anxiety
   C. Nurse pain assessment
   D. Support from others
   E. Culture
   F. Age

Copyright © 2018 Elsevier Canada, a division of Reed Elsevier Canada, Ltd.

10. The nurse needs certain information to assess the client's pain. Which of the following questions could you ask to help gather this information for the nurse?
    A. Where is the pain?
    B. How bad is the pain on a scale of 1–30?
    C. When did the pain start?
    D. Describe the pain.

11. Which of the following are safety measures used when the client is receiving strong pain medication?
    A. Keep hospital beds in the lowest position
    B. Provide assistance when the client is ambulating
    C. Keep bed rails up
    D. Check on the client every 10 to 15 minutes
    E. Provide a calm, quiet, darkened environment

12. Which of the following body responses may be signs and symptoms of pain?
    A. Nausea
    B. Increased pulse, respirations, and blood pressure
    C. Dry skin
    D. Sweating
    E. Vomiting

MULTIPLE CHOICE

Circle the correct answer.

13. The call bell should always be positioned:
    A. On the bed rail
    B. Attached to the pillow
    C. Within the client's reach
    D. On the arm of the chair

14. What type of pain is felt suddenly from injury, disease, trauma, or surgery?
    A. Persistent pain
    B. Severe pain
    C. Acute pain
    D. Mild pain

15. How long should you wait to perform procedures after pain medications are given?
    A. 5 minutes
    B. 10 minutes
    C. 30 minutes
    D. 60 minutes

16. What should you do if a client expresses an intention to leave the facility without the doctor's permission?
    A. Try to talk the client out of it
    B. Tell the nurse immediately
    C. Call the doctor to get permission
    D. Let the client leave as it is his or her choice

17. If you wish to locate an item in a client's closet, you should:
    A. Wait until the client is out of the room to search for it
    B. Tell the client that you must find the item and begin to search
    C. Ask the client for permission to look for the item
    D. Inform the nurse and have her look for the item

18. You are admitting a new client. Which of these situations should be reported to the nurse immediately?
    A. The client complains of pain and appears to be in distress
    B. The client cries and expresses a desire to go home
    C. The client has difficulty hearing you
    D. Both A and B

19. Mrs. Smith is being admitted to a facility. She wants a family member to stay with her during the admission process. What should you do?
    A. Tell the family member he or she must leave
    B. Tell the nurse
    C. Understand that this is a critical and emotional time for Mrs. Smith and her family and let the family member stay
    D. Address all questions to the family member because he or she can answer more quickly than Mrs. Smith can

Copyright © 2018 Elsevier Canada, a division of Reed Elsevier Canada, Ltd.

20. Which of the following tasks is a support worker's responsibility when a client is being discharged?
    A. Packing the client's belongings
    B. Teaching the client about a new diet
    C. Making an appointment with the doctor for the client
    D. Teaching the client about dressing changes

21. Which of the following statements about pain is true?
    A. Pain is easy to measure with objective assessments.
    B. Pain is different for each client.
    C. Pain means there is no damage to body tissue.
    D. Moaning signifies severe pain.

22. Which of the following statements describes persistent pain?
    A. Pain that lasts less than 6 months.
    B. Pain that may be constant or occur off and on
    C. Pain that eventually disappears at night
    D. Pain that is easily treated with medication

23. What type of pain occurs when a client with an amputated leg still feels pain in the missing limb?
    A. Acute
    B. Persistent
    C. Radiating
    D. Phantom

24. If a client is unable to fall asleep, is unable to stay asleep, or awakens easily and cannot fall back to sleep, the client has which of the following conditions?
    A. Sleep deprivation
    B. Insomnia
    C. Sleepwalking
    D. Emotional problems

MATCHING

Match the psychosocial task as described by Erikson's theory with the age range at which it occurs.

25. _____ Generativity versus stagnation
26. _____ Initiative versus guilt
27. _____ Identity versus role confusion
28. _____ Integrity versus despair
29. _____ Trust versus mistrust
30. _____ Competence versus inferiority
31. _____ Intimacy versus isolation
32. _____ Autonomy versus doubt

A. 6 to 12 years
B. 1 to 3 years
C. 20 to 40 years
D. 12 to 20 years
E. 3 to 6 years
F. 65+ years
G. 40 to 65 years
H. 0 to 1 year

Copyright © 2018 Elsevier Canada, a division of Reed Elsevier Canada, Ltd.

Match one of Maslow's hierarchy of needs with each of the words or phrases.

33. _____ Clothing

34. _____ Closeness

35. _____ Experiencing one's potential

36. _____ Opinion of self

37. _____ Protection from harm

A. Physical

B. Safety

C. Love and belonging

D. Self-esteem

E. E. Self-actualization

Match the definition to the term.

38. _____ Absence of mental or physical stress

39. _____ Directing the client's attention away from pain

40. _____ Creating an image in the mind and focusing on it

A. Guided imagery

B. Distraction

C. Relaxation

Match the comfort factors with the actions that the support worker can take to control these factors.

41. _____ Adjusting the thermostat in the room

42. _____ Turning lights down during rest periods

43. _____ Emptying bedpans and urinals promptly

44. _____ Opening windows and doors and turning on fans as the client desires

45. _____ Talking quietly to staff members

A. Temperature

B. Ventilation

C. Noise

D. Odours

E. Lighting

Match the type of pain with the correct description.

46. _____ Pain is felt at the site of tissue damage and in nearby areas.

47. _____ Pain is felt suddenly and lasts a short time.

48. _____ Pain is felt in a body part that is no longer there.

49. _____ Pain lasts longer than 6 months.

A. Acute pain

B. Persistent pain

C. Radiating pain

D. Phantom pain

Copyright © 2018 Elsevier Canada, a division of Reed Elsevier Canada, Ltd.

FILL IN THE BLANK

Indicate whether each of the words below is:

A. *A behaviour that is a sign or symptom of pain*

B. *A descriptive word related to pain*

50. _____ Aching

51. _____ Throbbing

52. _____ Groaning

53. _____ Restlessness

54. _____ Squeezing

55. _____ Knifelike

56. _____ Dull

57. _____ Irritability

58. _____ Quietness

FILL IN THE BLANKS

59. What type of pain is felt suddenly from injury, disease, trauma, or surgery?

   _____

60. How do these factors affect pain?

   a. Past experience _____

   b. Anxiety _____

   c. Rest and sleep _____

   d. Attention _____

   e. Value or meaning of pain _____

   f. Support from others _____

   g. Culture _____

   h. Age _____

Copyright © 2018 Elsevier Canada, a division of Reed Elsevier Canada, Ltd.

61. The nurse needs certain information to assess the client's pain. What questions could you ask to help gather this information for the nurse?

    a. Location _____

    _____

    b. Onset and duration _____

    _____

    c. Intensity _____

    _____

    d. Description _____

    _____

    e. Factors causing pain _____

    _____

    f. Vital signs _____

    _____

    g. Other signs and symptoms _____

    _____

62. Why are older clients at greater risk for undetected disease or injury?

    _____

63. The nurse asks you to assist with these measures to control pain. What is done with each one?

    a. Distraction _____

    _____

    b. Relaxation _____

    _____

    c. Guided imagery _____

    _____

64. When a client experiences pain, it cannot be seen, heard, felt, or smelled. How can you know the client has pain? _____

65. What are some ways you may be able to tell that an infant or young child has pain?

    _____

66. Ill or injured clients need to rest more often. How can you help them to get the rest needed?

    _____

    _____

67. What foods or liquids can help a person fall sleep?

    _____

68. How do the following factors affect sleep?
    a. Illness _____
    b. Nutrition _____
    c. Exercise at bedtime _____
    d. Environment _____
    e. Medications and alcohol _____
    f. Changes and stress _____
    g. Emotional problems _____

69. What can you do to the client's room to promote sleep?
    a. _____
    b. _____
    c. _____
    d. _____

70. What drinks should be avoided before going to bed?
    a. _____
    b. _____

71. List ways that a homelike environment can be provided in a long-term care facility.
    a. _____
    b. _____
    c. _____
    d. _____

72. Higher room temperatures will probably be needed by clients in these age groups.
    a. _____
    b. _____

73. Why are toilets in some health care facilities higher than standard toilets?
    a. _____
    b. _____

Copyright © 2018 Elsevier Canada, a division of Reed Elsevier Canada, Ltd.

LABELLING

Label each section of the pyramid with the basic need according to Maslow.

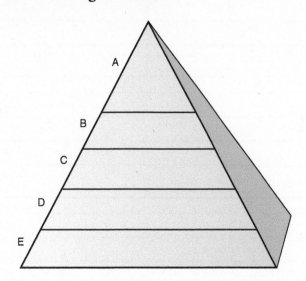

Match each section of the pyramid with the basic need according to Maslow

74. _____Self-esteem

75. _____Love and belonging

76. _____Physical

77. _____Self-actualization

78. _____Safety

Copyright © 2018 Elsevier Canada, a division of Reed Elsevier Canada, Ltd.

Medical Terminology

MULTIPLE CHOICE

Circle the word in each group that is spelled correctly.

1. Slow heart rate:
   A. Bradecardia
   B. Bradycardia
   C. Bradacordia
   D. Bradicardia

2. Difficulty urinating:
   A. Dysuria
   B. Dysurya
   C. Dysuira
   D. Disuria

3. Paralysis on one side of the body:
   A. Hemyplegia
   B. Hemaplegia
   C. Hemoplega
   D. Hemiplegia

4. Opening into the ileum:
   A. Illeostomy
   B. Ileostomy
   C. Ileastoma
   D. Illiostomy

5. Blue colour or condition:
   A. Cyonosis
   B. Cyinosis
   C. Cyanosis
   D. Cianosys

6. Opening into the trachea:
   A. Tracheastomy
   B. Trachiostomy
   C. Tracheostome
   D. Tracheostomy

7. Pain in a nerve:
   A. Neuralgia
   B. Neuroalgia
   C. Nourealgia
   D. Neurilegia

8. Examination of a joint with a scope:
   A. Arthoscope
   B. Arthroscopy
   C. Arethroscopy
   D. Artheroscope

9. Rapid breathing:
   A. Tachepnea
   B. Tachypinea
   C. Tachypnea
   D. Tachypnia

Copyright © 2018 Elsevier Canada, a division of Reed Elsevier Canada, Ltd.

10. Removal of the gallbladder:
    A.   Cholecystectomy
    B.   Cholcystectomy
    C.   Cholicystetomy
    D.   Cholecistectomy

MATCHING

Match the word with the correct definition.

11. Neuralgia	A. Painful or difficult urination
12. Gastrostomy	B. Inflammation of the kidneys
13. Cholecystectomy	C. Bluish colour
14. Dysuria	D. Caused by bacteria
15. Gastritis	E. Study of the skin
16. Enteritis	F. Incision into large intestine
17. Bacteriogenic	G. Instrument used to examine bronchi
18. Glossitis	H. Inflammation of the tongue
19. Cyanotic	I. Nerve pain
20. Dermatology	J. Examination of the rectum with an instrument
21. Oophorectomy	K. Excision (removal) of the gallbladder
22. Colostomy	L. Excision (removal) of an ovary
23. Nephritis	M. Incision into the stomach
24. Bronchoscope	N. Inflammation of the stomach
25. Proctoscopy	O. Inflammation of the intestine

Copyright © 2018 Elsevier Canada, a division of Reed Elsevier Canada, Ltd.

Match the prefix with the definition.

26. _____ auto-

27. _____ brady-

28. _____ circum-

29. _____ dys-

30. _____ ecto-

31. _____ leuk-

32. _____ macro-

33. _____ neo-

34. _____ supra-

35. _____ uni-

A.   Around

B.   White

C.   Self

D.   Large

E.   Outer, outside

F.   Slow

G.   Above, over

H.   One

I.   New

J.   Difficult, abnormal

Match each root word with the correct definition.

36. _____ aden(o)

37. _____ angi(o)

38. _____ bronch(o)

39. _____ crani(o)

40. _____ duoden(o)

41. _____ enter(o)

42. _____ gynec(o)

43. _____ mast(o)

44. _____ myel(o)

45. _____ py(o)

A.   Bronchus, bronchi

B.   Duodenum

C.   Women

D.   Spinal cord, bone marrow

E.   Pus

F.   Gland

G.   Mammary gland, breast

H.   Intestines

I.   Skull

J.   Vessel

Copyright © 2018 Elsevier Canada, a division of Reed Elsevier Canada, Ltd.

Match each suffix with the correct definition.

46. _____ -asis

47. _____ -genic

48. _____ -ism

49. _____ -oma

50. _____ -phasia

51. _____ -ptosis

52. _____ -plegia

53. _____ -megaly

54. _____ -scopy

55. _____ -stasis

A. Tumour

B. Falling, sagging, dropping, down

C. Enlargement

D. Paralysis

E. Examination using a scope

F. Condition, usually abnormal

G. Maintenance, maintaining a constant level

H. A condition

I. Speaking

J. Producing, causing

Match the following phrases or terms with the correct abbreviation.

56. _____ Abdomen

57. _____ Before meals

58. _____ After meals

59. _____ With

60. _____ Cancer

61. _____ Discontinue

62. _____ Lower left quadrant

63. _____ Every day

64. _____ Range of motion

A. c

B. d/c

C. QD

D. pc

E. ROM

F. CA

G. abd

H. LLQ

I. ac

Copyright © 2018 Elsevier Canada, a division of Reed Elsevier Canada, Ltd.

Match the following abbreviations with the correct word.

65. _____ s

66. _____ a.m.

67. _____ H₂O

68. _____ wt

69. _____ ht

70. _____ w/c

71. _____ stat

72. _____ O₂

73. _____ C

74. _____ bid

75. _____ CBR

76. _____ NPO

77. _____ prn

78. _____ qhs

79. _____ ROM

80. _____ RLQ

81. _____ SOB

82. _____ tid

83. _____ qid

84. _____ CPR

85. _____ LLQ

86. _____ VS

A. Weight

B. Twice a day

C. Nothing by mouth

D. Height

E. Three times a day

F. Complete bed rest

G. Wheelchair

H. Without

I. Centigrade

J. Every night at bedtime

K. Cardiopulmonary resuscitation

L. Morning

M. When necessary

N. Right lower quadrant

O. At once, immediately

P. Four times a day

Q. Left lower quadrant

R. Water

S. Shortness of breath

T. Oxygen

U. Vital signs

V. Range of motion

Copyright © 2018 Elsevier Canada, a division of Reed Elsevier Canada, Ltd.

Match the following terms with the correct definition.

87. _____ Hepatomegaly

88. _____ Hemiplegia

89. _____ Cholecystectomy

90. _____ Laparotomy

91. _____ Bradycardia

92. _____ Neuropathy

93. _____ Tachypnea

94. _____ Polyuria

95. _____ Pyorrhea

96. _____ Erythrocytopenia

97. _____ Leukocyte

98. _____ Bronchoscopy

99. _____ Encephalopathy

100. _____ Stomatitis

A.   Incision into the abdomen

B.   Disease of the nervous system

C.   Excessive urination

D.   Deficiency of red blood cells

E.   Slow heart rate

F.   Enlarged liver

G.   Excision (removal) of the gallbladder

H.   White blood cell

I.   A disease of the brain

J.   Discharge of pus

K.   Paralysis of one side of the body

L.   Rapid breathing

M.   Inflammation of the mouth

N.   Examination of the bronchi using a scope

Copyright © 2018 Elsevier Canada, a division of Reed Elsevier Canada, Ltd.

WORD SEARCH

For questions 101 to 113, write the correct term next to each abbreviation given. For questions 114 to 125, write the correct abbreviation next to the term given. Then find the answers (words and abbreviations) in the following puzzle.

101. s _____

102. am _____

103. CA _____

104. H_2O _____

105. gal _____

106. wt _____

107. ht _____

108. w/c _____

109. c _____

110. stat _____

111. O_2 _____

112. abd _____

113. post op _____

114. Twice a day _____

115. Complete bed rest _____

116. Nothing by mouth _____

117. When necessary _____

118. Every night at bedtime _____

119. Range of motion _____

120. Right lower quadrant _____

121. Shortness of breath _____

122. Three times a day _____

123. Four times a day _____

124. Left lower quadrant _____

125. Vital signs _____

```
N E U N I T N O C S I D R O E S S
U S R P R N A Q O A W I T H O L T
R T I O E M O D B A B E E Q L R
S A M L T C D A H H E I G H L T O
E T B U T A L L C O R V W E H L K
M O R N I N G L M Q B W E I G H T G
C X R I D C E M I S R R T Q L L A
A Y W A T N E R H O A R Y H S I E L
R G R T H R G B M M V S A T E L D Y L
E E L W E I M M P D I A T E V E O
E N P O S T O P E R A T I V E N
```

USING WORD ELEMENTS

The following words are made up of prefixes, root words, and suffixes. Identify each of the word elements using one of these methods:

Circle the prefixes in black, the root words in red, and the suffixes in blue.

OR

Highlight the prefixes in yellow, the root words in pink, and the suffixes in blue.

In the space following each word, define the word.

126. Hepatomegaly _____

    _____

127. Hemiplegia _____

    _____

128. Cholecystectomy _____

    _____

129. Laparotomy _____

    _____

130. Bradycardia _____

    _____

131. Neuropathy _____

    _____

132. Tachypnea _____

    _____

133. Polyuria _____

    _____

134. Pyorrhea _____

    _____

135. Dysphagia _____

136. Erythrocytopenia _____

137. Leukocyte _____

138. Bronchoscopy _____

139. Encephalopathy _____

    _____

140. Stomatitis _____

    _____

Copyright © 2018 Elsevier Canada, a division of Reed Elsevier Canada, Ltd.

Client Care: Planning, Processes, Reporting, and Recording

TRUE OR FALSE

The following statements apply to rules for recording. Circle T for true, or circle F for false.

1. **T** **F** Document in pencil.

2. **T** **F** Include the date whenever a new entry is made.

3. **T** **F** In written notes, all writing must be legible and *neat*.

4. **T** **F** Use any abbreviations needed to shorten an entry.

5. **T** **F** Use correct spelling, grammar, and punctuation.

6. **T** **F** For written documentation, use an eraser or correction fluid if you make an error.

7. **T** **F** Sign all entries with your name and title as required by your agency.

8. **T** **F** Skip lines between recorded entries.

9. **T** **F** Document what you or others did or observed.

10. **T** **F** Document all care and treatments early in the shift before beginning work.

11. **T** **F** Document your observations, interpretations, and judgements.

12. **T** **F** Document in a logical and sequential manner.

13. **T** **F** Avoid terms with more than one meaning.

14. **T** **F** Paraphrase the client's words to make the meaning more understandable.

15. **T** **F** Document any changes from normal or changes in the client's condition.

16. **T   F**   Repeated complaints of pain can be omitted when documenting.

17. **T   F**   Document safety measures used in caring for the client.

18. **T   F**   Objective data are things a client reports that you cannot observe by using your senses.

19. **T   F**   Subjective data are pieces of information you can obtain about a client using your senses.

20. **T   F**   When you document in the chart, you sign your name and write your title as per agency policy after each entry.

MULTIPLE RESPONSE

From the list below, choose all of the correct answers.

21. What are the four senses you use to obtain information about a client?
    A.   Smell
    B.   Hearing
    C.   Touch
    D.   Instinct
    E.   Sight

22. Which of the following basic observations will give you information about a client?
    A.   ADLs
    B.   Appetite
    C.   Pain
    D.   Respirations
    E.   Skin condition
    F.   Ability to respond

23. What basic observations can you make to determine a client's ability to respond?
    A.   The client can state his or her name, the time, and the location
    B.   The client can speak clearly
    C.   The client can follow directions
    D.   The family can answer questions
    E.   The client is easy to rouse
    F.   The client responds correctly to questions

24. What observations will help to determine whether a client is moving appropriately?
    A.   The client can squeeze your fingers with each hand
    B.   The client can move his or her arms and legs
    C.   The client's movements are shaky or jerky
    D.   The client can ambulate without assistance

25. What observations should be made about a client's respirations?
    A.   Do both sides of the client's chest rise and fall with respirations?
    B.   Is the client's breathing noisy?
    C.   Does the client complain of difficulty breathing?
    D.   Does the client complain of gas?
    E.   What is the amount and colour of sputum?
    F.   What is the frequency of the client's cough? Is it dry or productive?

26. What observations should be made about the skin?
    A.   Is the skin pale or flushed?
    B.   Is the skin moist or dry?
    C.   Is the skin intact?
    D.   Are bruises present? Where?
    E.   Is the abdomen firm or soft?
    F.   Does the client complain of itching?

27. What observations are important to determine how the bowels and bladder are functioning?
    A.   Amount, colour, and consistency of stool
    B.   Colour of the lips and nail beds
    C.   Frequency of bowel movements
    D.   Pain or difficulty urinating
    E.   Client's control of the passage of urine
    F.   Frequency of urination

28. When reporting to the nurse, you should do which of the following?
    A. Report what you observed and did yourself
    B. Report what other support workers did
    C. Report any changes in the client's condition.
    D. Report promptly, thoroughly, and accurately
    E. Report only at the end of your shift

MULTIPLE CHOICE

Circle the correct answer.

29. What information is included on the graphic sheet?
    A. Bowel sounds
    B. Temperature, pulse, and respirations
    C. Complaints of pain
    D. Amount of food consumed

30. What statement about electronic documentation is correct?
    A. You are able to use all types of abbreviations.
    B. All spelling errors are automatically corrected.
    C. In general, staff can take tablets home to document on their own time.
    D. It requires individual entries using a personal identification number (PIN) or code.

31. Which of these is a question about an activity of daily living?
    A. Can the client perform personal care without help?
    B. How much food on the tray did the client eat?
    C. What is the frequency of the client's bowel movements?
    D. Can the client move his or her arms and legs?

32. When should the support worker contact the supervisor?
    A. When the pharmacy delivers the client's medications to the house.
    B. When you believe the client's safety is at risk.
    C. The support worker should provide the supervisor with hourly updates.
    D. After completion of a procedure.

Copyright © 2018 Elsevier Canada, a division of Reed Elsevier Canada, Ltd.

MATCHING

Match the following descriptions with one of the key terms related to communication.

33. _____ Identification of a disease or condition by a doctor

34. _____ Determining whether the goals in the care plan have been met

35. _____ Description of a health problem that can be treated by nursing measures

36. _____ Written guide that gives direction about the care and services a client should receive

37. _____ Method used by nurses to plan and deliver nursing care

38. _____ Action taken by a nursing team member to help the client reach a goal

A. Client care plan

B. Nursing diagnosis

C. Nursing intervention

D. Care planning process

E. Medical diagnosis

F. Evaluation

Copyright © 2018 Elsevier Canada, a division of Reed Elsevier Canada, Ltd.

Match the following time with the corresponding time using the 24-hour clock.

39. _____ 8:45 a.m.

40. _____ 4:00 p.m.

41. _____ 11:59 p.m.

42. _____ 12:30 a.m.

43. _____ 9:50 p.m.

44. _____ midnight

45. _____ 6:30 a.m.

46. _____ 10:00 p.m.

47. _____ 1:30 p.m.

48. _____ 7:30 p.m.

49. _____ 3:30 p.m.

50. _____ 2:45 p.m.

A.   0030 hr

B.   2400 or 0000 hr

C.   2200 hr

D.   0630 hr

E.   1930 hr

F.   1530 hr

G.   0845 hr

H.   2359 hr

I.   1445 hr

J.   1330 hr

K.   2150 hr

L.   1600 hr

Copyright © 2018 Elsevier Canada, a division of Reed Elsevier Canada, Ltd.

FILL IN THE BLANKS

The following words or phrases are either subjective (S) or objective (O) data. Fill in the blank with either an S or an O.

51. _____ Sleepy

52. _____ Chest pain

53. _____ Cool skin

54. _____ Bruises

55. _____ Difficulty breathing

56. _____ Gas pain

57. _____ Pain when urinating

58. _____ Productive cough

59. _____ Breath has a fruity odour

60. _____ Rapid pulse and shallow breathing

61. _____ Mr. Khan states that he is cold

62. _____ Mary has red hair

63. _____ Mrs. Smith says she has pain in her right shoulder

64. _____ Temperature 37.6°C (99.6°F), pulse 72, respirations 16

65. _____ Mr. Kallio ate all of his breakfast

66. _____ Mrs. Foster says she is anxious about having surgery

Copyright © 2018 Elsevier Canada, a division of Reed Elsevier Canada, Ltd.

CHAPTER 15

Measuring Height, Weight, and Vital Signs

TRUE OR FALSE

Circle T for true, or circle F for false.

1. **T** **F** A handheld electronic thermometer is stored in a storage box.

2. **T** **F** Systole is the period of time when the heart muscle is relaxed.

3. **T** **F** Bradycardia is a rapid heart rate.

4. **T** **F** Blood pressure is normally measured in the brachial artery.

5. **T** **F** If you are unsure you have taken an accurate blood pressure reading, you should take off the cuff and try again in 30 to 60 seconds.

6. **T** **F** The systolic pressure is the lower pressure.

7. **T** **F** Respiratory rates vary with age.

8. **T** **F** A tympanic membrane thermometer is inserted into the ear to measure body temperature.

9. **T** **F** An axillary temperature taken with a thermometer can take up to 2 minutes to register accurately.

10. **T** **F** The earpieces and diaphragm on a stethoscope should never be cleaned with alcohol wipes.

11. **T** **F** Rhythm and force are characteristics of a pulse.

12. **T** **F** You should avoid using your thumb to take a pulse because you could mistake the pulse in your thumb for the client's pulse.

13. **T** **F** Blood pressure increases with age, up to adulthood.

14. **T** **F** Women usually have higher blood pressures than men.

15. **T** **F** The lower the blood volume, the lower the blood pressure.

16. **T** **F** Stress decreases blood pressure.

17. **T** **F** Blood pressure is higher in overweight people.

Copyright © 2018 Elsevier Canada, a division of Reed Elsevier Canada, Ltd.

73

18. **T   F**   Blood pressure tends to be lower among people of South Asian, Aboriginal, and African descent.

19. **T   F**   Smoking increases blood pressure.

20. **T   F**   Normal newborn respirations are 30–60 respirations/minute.

21. **T   F**   25–32 respirations/minute is normal for a healthy adult.

MULTIPLE RESPONSE

From the list below, choose all of the correct answers.

22. When would you expect vital signs to be measured?
    A. During physical examinations
    B. When a person is admitted to a facility
    C. Once a day for hospital patients
    D. Before and after surgery
    E. Before a fall or other injury
    F. When medications are taken that affect the respiratory or circulatory system
    G. Whenever the client complains of pain, dizziness, light-headedness, shortness of breath, rapid heart rate, or not feeling well
    H. As stated in the care plan (usually daily or weekly)

23. The temperature should not be taken orally if the client:
    A. Is conscious
    B. Has had surgery or an injury to the face, neck, nose, or mouth
    C. Has a nasogastric tube
    D. Is delirious, restless, confused, or disoriented
    E. Is paralyzed on one side of the body
    F. Has a sore mouth
    G. Has a convulsive disorder
    H. Is receiving oxygen therapy

24. Which of the following factors can affect the pulse rate?
    A. Elevated body temperature
    B. Exercise
    C. Pain
    D. Position change
    E. Caffeine
    F. Medications

25. When you are taking a client's blood pressure, which of the following guidelines should you follow?
    A. Take blood pressure on an arm with an IV infusion, cast, or dialysis access site; an injured arm; or on the side where the client has had breast surgery.
    B. Let the client rest for 10 to 20 minutes first.
    C. Measure blood pressure with the client standing.
    D. Use the correct-sized blood pressure cuff.
    E. Apply the cuff over the shirt sleeve.
    F. Make sure the cuff is snug.
    G. Place the diaphragm of the stethoscope firmly over the artery.
    H. Have the manometer clearly visible.
    I. The first sound is the diastolic pressure.
    J. Wait 5–10 seconds before repeating the measurement.

MULTIPLE CHOICE

Circle the correct answer.

26. Why is it important to keep a record of previous vital signs?
    A. The support worker can prove that they were taken.
    B. The doctor or nurse can compare each measurement.
    C. The client's family can check to see if the care is being given.
    D. The support worker can see if the readings obtained are accurate compared with others.

Copyright © 2018 Elsevier Canada, a division of Reed Elsevier Canada, Ltd.

27. When you take the vital signs and they have changed from a previous measurement, what should you do?
    A. Record the results promptly in the client's record.
    B. Circle the changes in red.
    C. Report the changes to the nurse promptly.
    D. Take them again in 15 minutes.

28. Which of these statements about electronic thermometers is not true?
    A. The temperature display is easily read.
    B. If the probe is broken, the client could swallow mercury.
    C. The temperature is rapidly measured.
    D. Disposable covers reduce the possibility of spreading infection.

29. If the client is smoking and you need to take an oral temperature, what should you do?
    A. Provide oral hygiene first.
    B. Wait 15 minutes to take the temperature.
    C. Take a rectal temperature instead.
    D. Wait 45 minutes to take the temperature.

30. For how long should you take an irregular pulse?
    A. 30 seconds
    B. 2 minutes
    C. 5 minutes
    D. 1 full minute

31. When assessing the client's pulse, which of the following pulse rates should be reported to the nurse immediately?
    A. 72
    B. 50
    C. 60
    D. 98

32. You are assigned to take the blood pressure of several clients. Which of these measurements should you report immediately?
    A. 140/80
    B. 138/90
    C. 150/110
    D. 96/70

33. What best describes a pulse oximeter? It is a device that:
    A. Measures the client's pulse and blood pressure
    B. Measures the oxygen level in the blood and pulse
    C. Assesses the client's response to pain
    D. Measures the pH level of the client's blood

Copyright © 2018 Elsevier Canada, a division of Reed Elsevier Canada, Ltd.

MATCHING

Match the parts of the stethoscope as indicated in the diagram.

34. _____ Diaphragm

35. _____ Bell

36. _____ Earpieces

37. _____ Binaurals

38. _____ Rubber or plastic tubing

39. _____ Chest piece

Copyright © 2018 Elsevier Canada, a division of Reed Elsevier Canada, Ltd.

Match the site of the temperature to the normal range for that site.

40. _____ Oral

41. _____ Axillary

42. _____ Tympanic membrane

A. 35.5 to 37.5°C

B. 34.7 to 37.3°C

C. 35.8 to 38.0°C

Match the name of the pulse site to where you would find the pulse on the body.

43. Temporal

44. Carotid

45. Brachial

46. Radial

47. Femoral

48. Popliteal

49. Dorsalis pedis

50. Apical

A. Inside the elbows

B. Ankles

C. Top of inner thighs

D. Chest

E. Sides of the neck

F. Knees

G. Sides of the head

H. Wrists

Match the normal pulse ranges with the correct age group.

51. 80 to 180

52. 70 to 110

53. 80 to 120

54. 60 to 100

A. 6 to 12 years

B. 2 to 6 years

C. Birth to 1 year

D. 12 years and older

Copyright © 2018 Elsevier Canada, a division of Reed Elsevier Canada, Ltd.

Match the definition with the correct term.

55. Taking the apical and radial pulses at the same time

56. Amount of force exerted against the walls of an artery by the blood

57. Condition in which the systolic blood pressure is below 90 mm Hg and the diastolic pressure is below 60 mm Hg

58. Instrument used to listen to the sounds produced by the heart, lungs, and other body organs

59. A slow heart rate; rate is less than 60 beats per minute

60. Act of breathing air into and out of the lungs

61. Persistent blood pressure measurements above the normal systolic

62. Rapid heart rate; rate is over 100 beats per minute

63. Period of heart muscle relaxation

64. Beat of the heart felt at an artery as a wave of blood passes through the artery

65. Instrument used to measure blood pressure

66. Temperature, pulse, respirations, and blood pressure *(two words)*

67. Period of heart muscle contraction

A. Respiration

B. Tachycardia

C. Apical radial pulse

D. Diastole

E. Hypertension

F. Blood pressure

G. Bradycardia

H. Systole

I. Hypotension

J. Pulse

K. Vital signs

L. Stethoscope

M. Sphygmomanometer

Copyright © 2018 Elsevier Canada, a division of Reed Elsevier Canada, Ltd.

FILL IN THE BLANKS

Identify whether the following words are used when discussing:

A. **Pulse**
B. **Blood pressure**

68. _____ Radial

69. _____ Bradycardia

70. _____ Hypertension

71. _____ Systole

72. _____ Hypotension

73. _____ Diastole

74. _____ Apical

75. _____ Tachycardia

76. For how long is an axillary temperature taken with a thermometer?

_____

77. Why are the earpieces and diaphragm on a stethoscope cleaned with alcohol wipes before and after use?

_____

78. How can you prevent noise when you are using a stethoscope?

_____

79. When you are measuring the pulse, what two characteristics of the pulse should be noted in addition to the rate?

_____

80. Why do you keep your fingers or stethoscope in place after you count the pulse and while you count the respirations?

_____

Copyright © 2018 Elsevier Canada, a division of Reed Elsevier Canada, Ltd.

81. How do these factors affect the blood pressure?

    a. Age _____

    b. Gender _____

    c. Blood volume _____

    d. Stress _____

    e. Pain _____

    f. Exercise _____

    g. Weight _____

    h. Race _____

    i. Diet _____

    j. Drugs _____

    k. Position _____

    l. Smoking _____

    m. Alcohol _____

82. If a client cannot stand up to have his or her height measured, what procedure will help you to gather this information?

    _____

    _____

    _____

83. Why do you ensure your client has voided before you weigh him or her?

    _____

    _____

84. The height or length of a young child is taken from the _____ to the _____.

85. What is the normal respiratory rate for the following ages?

    a. Newborn _____

    b. 10 years _____

    c. 2 years _____

    d. Healthy adult _____

Copyright © 2018 Elsevier Canada, a division of Reed Elsevier Canada, Ltd.

LABELLING

86. Fill in the following drawings so that the dials show the correct blood pressures.
    a.   168/102
    b.   104/68

87. Fill in the following drawings so that the mercury columns show the correct blood pressure.
    a.   152/86
    b.   198/110

Copyright © 2018 Elsevier Canada, a division of Reed Elsevier Canada, Ltd.

CROSSWORD

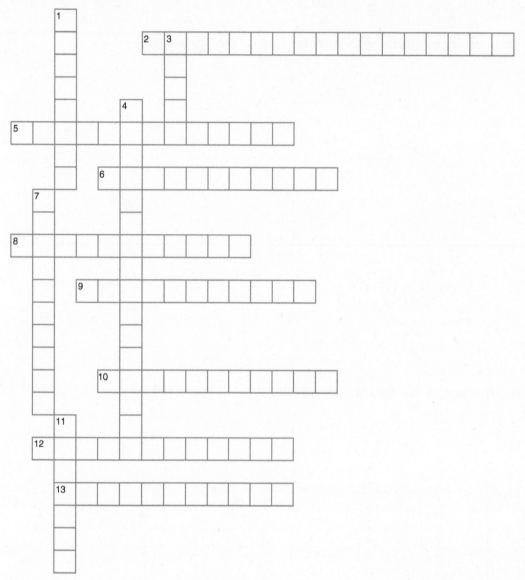

Across

2. Taking the apical and radial pulses at the same time *(3 words)*
5. Amount of force exerted against the walls of an artery by the blood *(2 words)*
6. Condition in which the systolic blood pressure is below 90 mm Hg and the diastolic pressure is below 60 mm Hg
8. Instrument used to listen to the sounds produced by the heart, lungs, and other body organs
9. A slow heart rate; rate is less than 60 beats per minute
10. Act of breathing air into and out of the lungs
12. Persistent blood pressure measurements above the normal systolic (140 mm Hg) or diastolic (90 mm Hg) pressures
13. Rapid heart rate; heart rate is over 100 beats per minute

Down

1. Period of heart muscle relaxation
3. Beat of the heart felt at an artery as a wave of blood passes through the artery
4. Instrument used to measure blood pressure
7. Temperature, pulse, respirations, and blood pressure *(2 words)*
11. Period of heart muscle contraction

Copyright © 2018 Elsevier Canada, a division of Reed Elsevier Canada, Ltd.

Abuse Awareness

TRUE OR FALSE

Circle T for true, or circle F for false.

1. T F Usually, the time between abusive events gradually shortens.

2. T F More men than women are abused by spouses.

3. T F People who are abused often deny the abuse.

4. T F Slapping a child is not considered abuse.

5. T F Emotional and physical abuse are the most common types of abuse of older adults.

6. T F Ageism is another cause of abuse.

7. T F Failing to provide privacy is not a form of abuse.

8. T F Changes in mental function can cause someone to become sexually abusive.

9. T F Masturbation may be the result of urinary problems in a confused client.

10. T F The best way to handle a client who is masturbating in public is to tell the client to stop.

11. T F You are legally responsible to report child abuse and (in some jurisdictions) abuse within facilities.

12. T F Sexual harassment is not considered sexual abuse.

13. T F Abuse is usually triggered by an event related to the victim.

14. T F People who were abused as children are not likely to abuse their own children because they know what it was like.

15. T F In most provinces, you do not have to report abuse of older adults to a public authority if it occurs in home care settings.

Copyright © 2018 Elsevier Canada, a division of Reed Elsevier Canada, Ltd.

16. **T   F**   If you suspect abuse, you should document your findings privately, without making assumptions. Keep all of your notes for future reference.

17. **T   F**   For suspected child abuse, do not rely on your supervisor to report your observations to child protection authorities.

MULTIPLE RESPONSE

From the list below, choose all of the correct answers.

18. The three phases in the cycle of abuse are:
    A.   Tension-building
    B.   Trust-building
    C.   Abuse
    D.   Denial
    E.   Bargaining
    F.   Honeymoon

19. A person is more likely to be abusive if he or she:
    A.   Holds a responsible job
    B.   Has problems with alcohol or drugs
    C.   Lives alone
    D.   Has a mental health disorder or severe personality flaws
    E.   Was abused as a child
    F.   Is going through a period of high stress

20. Certain situations increase the risk of child abuse. They are:
    A.   Family crisis
    B.   Nonbiological or temporary caregivers in the home
    C.   Isolation
    D.   Caring for children with special needs
    E.   Extremely high or low intelligence

21. Why do abused older adults choose not to complain about the abuse?
    A.   They do not know they are being abused.
    B.   They would rather find a lawyer and sue the abuser in court.
    C.   They may fear the abuser.
    D.   They may not know where or how to get help.
    E.   They may fear being forced to move into a facility if the abuser is the primary caregiver.
    F.   They may have physical or mental health disabilities that prevent them from reporting.

22. Examples of how workers might abuse clients in a facility or home are:
    A.   Using restraints inappropriately
    B.   Handling the client roughly
    C.   Isolating the client
    D.   Stealing from the client
    E.   Not reviewing the care plan regularly
    F.   Not responding to a call for help
    G.   Not checking on the client for long periods of time
    H.   Leaving the client in soiled linen or clothes

23. What are some examples of abuse that a support worker may encounter from clients?
    A.   Swearing, name-calling, and using racial or cultural slurs
    B.   Threats
    C.   Denial of meal breaks, drinking water, bathroom use, or handwashing facilities
    D.   Hitting, pushing, kicking, spitting, biting, pinching, or other physical attacks
    E.   Taking too long to eat meals
    F.   Inappropriate touching, sexual assault or harassment

Copyright © 2018 Elsevier Canada, a division of Reed Elsevier Canada, Ltd.

24. People at highest risk for abuse include:
    A. Older adults cared for by people with substance abuse problems
    B. Older adults who are financially stable
    C. Older adults who are unable to leave their homes
    D. Older adults with disabilities who are dependent on their caregivers
    E. Older adults with dementia

25. People at greatest risk for marginalization include those who:
    A. Work in the sex-trade industry
    B. Have a physical or intellectual disability
    C. Are assertive in nature
    D. Belong to a visible-minority group
    E. Are college graduates
    F. Are substance abusers
    G. Cannot speak an official language
    H. Have a mental health disorder

26. What can you do when a client is being abusive?
    A. Stay calm and stand up so as not to be dominated by the client, but stand far enough away so that the person cannot reach you.
    B. Position yourself close to a door, and note the location of call bells, alarms, and other security devices.
    C. Keep your hands free, but do not touch the client.
    D. Listen to the client. Restate what the person says in your own words.
    E. Raise your voice to show your dominance and control over the client.
    F. Tell the client you will get your supervisor to speak to him. If you cannot leave the room, sound the call bell, alarm, or other security device.
    G. If you are at a client's home and think you are in danger, leave the house immediately. Go to a safe place, and call your supervisor.
    H. If you are at a client's home, do not leave the client alone. Stay and reason with the client.

MULTIPLE CHOICE

Circle the correct answer.

27. If you suspect a client is being abused, you should:
    A. Call the police
    B. Talk to the family
    C. Report it to the nurse in charge
    D. Talk to the client being abused

28. If you are dealing with an agitated or aggressive client, which of these measures would be most helpful?
    A. Talking to the client in a calm manner
    B. Placing your hand on the client's arm to prevent injury
    C. Closing the door so that other people are not upset
    D. Promising the client you will not tell anyone else about her behaviour

29. During the "honeymoon phase" of the cycle of abuse:
    A. The abuser begins to get moodier and stressed
    B. The abuse can escalate easily even if unprovoked
    C. The abuser often blames the victim for the abuse
    D. The abuser is very apologetic for what happened

30. Mrs. Jones is not allowed to go to the bank. Her son insists on handling all of her finances. This is an example of:
    A. Neglect
    B. Physical abuse
    C. Financial abuse
    D. Sexual abuse

31. Mrs. Jones's son insists on changing his mother's incontinence briefs. This might be a sign of:
    A. Neglect
    B. Physical abuse
    C. Financial abuse
    D. Sexual abuse

Copyright © 2018 Elsevier Canada, a division of Reed Elsevier Canada, Ltd.

32. Mrs. Verbrugghe cannot speak English. Her son refuses to translate things for her, especially legal documents, such as the deed to her house. This might be a sign of:
    A. Neglect
    B. Physical abuse
    C. Financial abuse
    D. Sexual abuse

33. You are meeting your home care client, Mrs. Yil, for the first time in her home. While talking to her, you notice that she is very groggy, slurring her words, and smells of alcohol. What should you do first?
    A. Offer her coffee
    B. Notify your supervisor and ask what to do
    C. Inform the client that the nurse will come to her house to assess her
    D. Ask her if you should come back another time when she is more awake

34. You have been supporting Mrs. Yil for several weeks. During that time, you have noticed that she is very quiet whenever her daughter comes to visit her. You suspect abuse but cannot prove it. What should you do?
    A. Ignore it. They could just be having a bad day.
    B. Ask Mrs. Yil's daughter if she has noticed how quiet her mother is
    C. Telephone the police and make a complaint
    D. Discuss this situation with your supervisor

35. Miss Keys scratches and punches when it is time for her shower. What should you do?
    A. Stay calm and protect yourself
    B. Refuse to bathe Miss Keys
    C. Use silence and ignore her behaviour
    D. Hold her hands until she calms down.

36. When a client is angry and demanding, it is important to:
    A. Walk away and return in 1 hour
    B. Ignore the client until her behaviour improves
    C. Treat the person with respect and dignity
    D. Tell the client how irritating she is to the staff

37. A term used to describe infants, babies, or children who are below the norms for body weight, growth, or cognitive development is:
    A. Neglected
    B. Failure to thrive
    C. Refusal to grow
    D. Idiopathic weight challenge

MATCHING

Match each example with the letter that corresponds to the abuse type.
A. Neglect
B. Sexual abuse
C. Emotional abuse
D. Financial abuse
E. Physical abuse

38. _____ The person has physical injuries (e.g., burns, bumps, cuts, bruises, etc.).

39. _____ The person's behaviour changes when the caregiver (i.e., the potential abuser) leaves or enters the room.

40. _____ Medications are not purchased.

41. _____ The caregiver insists on being present or within hearing distance of all conversations.

42. _____ New injuries appear while older ones are still healing.

Copyright © 2018 Elsevier Canada, a division of Reed Elsevier Canada, Ltd.

43. _____ The person has an intense fear of bathing or perineal care.

44. _____ Personal hygiene is poor (e.g., ingrown nails, untreated sores, matted hair).

45. _____ The person's living conditions are unsafe, unclean, or inadequate.

46. _____ The person has irritation or injury of the thighs, perineum, or breasts.

47. _____ The person has many unpaid bills.

48. _____ The person has signs of poor nutrition and fluid intake (e.g., weight loss, sunken eyes, dry skin).

49. _____ The person may ask for permission to write cheques or spend money.

50. _____ The caregiver often complains about the client.

Match the correct terms with their definitions.

51. _____ Failure to meet basic needs

52. _____ Misuse of a client's money

53. _____ Force or violence that causes injury

54. _____ Unwanted sexual activity

55. _____ Words or actions that inflict mental harm

A. Sexual abuse

B. Physical abuse

C. Emotional abuse

D. Financial abuse

E. Neglect

Match the different forms of client abuse with the appropriate description.

56. _____ Threatening punishment or deprival of needs

57. _____ Inflicting punishment on the body

58. _____ Kissing, inappropriately touching, or fondling a child

59. _____ Spending a person's money without consent

60. _____ Providing care against a client's wishes

A. Physical

B. Violation of rights

C. Sexual

D. Financial

E. Emotional

Copyright © 2018 Elsevier Canada, a division of Reed Elsevier Canada, Ltd.

FILL IN THE BLANK

61. Give three signs/symptoms of each type of abuse.

Physical abuse

a. _____

b. _____

c. _____

Sexual abuse

a. _____

b. _____

c. _____

Emotional abuse

a. _____

b. _____

c. _____

Financial abuse

a. _____

b. _____

c. _____

Neglect

a. _____

b. _____

c. _____

Copyright © 2018 Elsevier Canada, a division of Reed Elsevier Canada, Ltd.

Body Structure and Function

TRUE OR FALSE

Circle T for true, or circle F for false.

1. **T** **F** The skin is the body's first line of defence against disease.

2. **T** **F** The optic nerve is found in the ear.

3. **T** **F** The immune system is made up of red blood cells.

4. **T** **F** The tympanic membrane is found in the ear.

5. **T** **F** Fingernails and toenails are part of the integumentary system.

6. **T** **F** The peripheral nervous system is made up of the brain and spinal cord.

7. **T** **F** The parasympathetic nervous system is responsible for flight, fright, or fight.

8. **T** **F** Bones are dead.

9. **T** **F** A function of the muscular system is to provide the body with heat.

10. **T** **F** The function of the urinary system is to remove waste products from the blood.

11. **T** **F** The process of cell division is called *mitosis*.

12. **T** **F** The ball-and-socket joint allows movement in all directions.

13. **T** **F** The hinge joint allows turning from side to side.

14. **T** **F** The pivot joint allows movement in one direction.

15. **T** **F** The pathways that conduct messages to and from the brain are contained in the spinal cord.

16. **T** **F** The small bones in the middle ear are called the *malleus*, *incus*, and *anvil*.

17. **T**   **F**   The function of the lungs is to allow respiration.

18. **T**   **F**   Urine is made up of waste products filtered out of the liver.

19. **T**   **F**   The master gland of the endocrine system is the pituitary gland.

20. **T**   **F**   The major function of the thyroid gland is to regulate calcium.

21. **T**   **F**   Glucocorticoids regulate the metabolism of carbohydrates.

22. **T**   **F**   Passive immunity is a natural process of developing antibodies within the body.

23. **T**   **F**   Cartilage is connective tissue that prevents bone ends from rubbing together.

24. **T**   **F**   Capillaries are the largest diameter blood vessels.

25. **T**   **F**   Chemical digestion is the act of chewing food.

MULTIPLE RESPONSE

From the list below, choose all of the correct answers.

26. What are the basic structures of the cell?
    A. Cell membrane
    B. Nucleus
    C. Pleura
    D. Cytoplasm
    E. Synovial fluid

27. Which of the following are the structures that make up the circulatory system?
    A. Blood
    B. Kidney
    C. Heart
    D. Vessels
    E. Spinal cord

28. Specialized connective tissue includes:
    A. Blood
    B. Bone
    C. Muscle
    D. Adipose
    E. Dense fibrous
    F. Nerve

29. The purpose of adipose tissue includes:
    A. Supplies energy to surrounding cells
    B. Assists in draining internal fluids
    C. Acts as a cushion to the body
    D. Supports surrounding structures
    E. Transports hormones to target organs
    F. Aids in body temperature regulation

30. Types of bones include:
    A. Flat bones
    B. Short bones
    C. Irregular bones
    D. Cartilage
    E. Long bones
    F. Spinal bones
    G. Sesamoid bones

MULTIPLE CHOICE

Circle the correct answer.

31. What is the name of the body function that burns food for heat and energy?
    A. Metabolism
    B. Digestion
    C. Peristalsis
    D. Urination

32. The urinary system consists of:
    A. 2 kidneys, 2 ureters, 2 urethras, 2 bladders
    B. 2 kidneys, 1 bladder, 1 ureter, 1 urethra
    C. Urethra and bladder only
    D. 2 kidneys, 2 ureters, 1 bladder, 1 urethra

33. Each system of the body is composed of:
    A. Cells, tissues, and bones
    B. Tissues, organs, and muscles
    C. Bones, muscles, and tissues
    D. Cells, tissues, and organs

Copyright © 2018 Elsevier Canada, a division of Reed Elsevier Canada, Ltd.

34. Smooth muscles may be found in the:
    A. Arms and legs
    B. Body track
    C. Digestive tract
    D. Head and neck

35. Which statement is true about cardiac muscle?
    A. It is classified as voluntary muscle
    B. Is found only in the heart
    C. It is used to create body heat
    D. It is found in the dorsal cavity

36. Which statement about the integumentary system is true?
    A. Consists of all four types of tissues working together
    B. The epidermis is the innermost layer of the skin
    C. The epidermis contains a vast supply of blood vessels
    D. Dead cells of the epidermis contain pigment

37. The middle layer of the skin is called the:
    A. Epidermis
    B. Dermis
    C. Subcutaneous
    D. Fat

38. An example of a hinge joint is the:
    A. Shoulder
    B. Knuckles at the base of the fingers
    C. Wrist
    D. Knee

39. Tendons connect:
    A. Muscles to muscles
    B. Nerve cells to muscles
    C. Bone to bone
    D. Muscles to bones

40. What type of blood vessel carries blood away from the heart?
    A. Artery
    B. Vein
    C. Vena cava
    D. Capillary

41. The cerebellum:
    A. Is also called the brain stem
    B. Controls the body's senses
    C. Regulates and controls body movement
    D. Is considered the largest part of the brain

42. The highest functions of the brain take place in the:
    A. Cerebral cortex
    B. Medulla
    C. Brain stem
    D. Spinal nerve

43. The endocrine glands secrete substances called:
    A. Hormones
    B. Mucus
    C. Semen
    D. Insulin

44. What is the major function of the thyroid gland?
    A. Regulates growth
    B. Prevents excessive loss of fluids
    C. Regulates metabolism
    D. Regulates calcium use by the body

45. Besides serving as the organ of hearing, the ear is involved with:
    A. Balance
    B. Regulating body movements
    C. Controlling involuntary muscles
    D. Smoothness of body movements

Copyright © 2018 Elsevier Canada, a division of Reed Elsevier Canada, Ltd.

MATCHING

Match the following statements with the correct terms.

46. _____ Blood vessel that carries blood away from the heart

47. _____ Blood vessel that carries blood back to the heart

48. _____ Tiny blood vessel that allows food, oxygen, and other substances to pass to the cells

49. _____ Basic unit of body structure

50. _____ Group of cells with the same function

51. _____ Group of tissues with the same function

52. _____ Organs that work together to perform special functions

53. _____ Process of physically and chemically breaking down food so it can be absorbed for use by the cells of the body

54. _____ Muscle contractions in the digestive system that move food through the alimentary canal

55. _____ Burning of food by the cells to produce heat and energy

A. Artery

B. Capillary

C. Cell

D. Digestion

E. Metabolism

F. Organ

G. Peristalsis

H. System

I. Tissue

J. Vein

Match the four basic types of tissue with their functions.

56. _____ Epithelial tissue

57. _____ Connective tissue

58. _____ Muscle tissue

59. _____ Nerve tissue

A. Anchors, connects, and supports other body tissues

B. Relays information to and from the brain and throughout the body

C. Allows the body to move by stretching and contracting

D. Covers internal and external body surfaces

Copyright © 2018 Elsevier Canada, a division of Reed Elsevier Canada, Ltd.

Match the bone with the correct description of what the bone does.

60. _____ Long bones

61. _____ Short bones

62. _____ Flat bones

63. _____ Irregular bones

A. Allow skill and ease in movement

B. Protect the organs

C. Bear the weight of the body

D. Allow various degrees of movement and flexibility

Match the following statements with one of the terms related to the digestive and urinary systems.

64. _____ Structure that adds digestive juices to chyme

65. _____ Semi-liquid food mixture formed in stomach

66. _____ Portion of the gastrointestinal tract that absorbs food

67. _____ Portion of the gastrointestinal tract that absorbs water

68. _____ Produces digestive juices

69. _____ Produces bile

70. _____ Basic working unit of the kidney

71. _____ Hollow muscular sac that stores urine

72. _____ Structure that allows urine to pass from the bladder

73. _____ Opening from the bladder at the end of the urethra

74. _____ Bean-shaped structure that produces urine

75. _____ Moistens food particles in the mouth

A. Bladder

B. Chyme

C. Colon

D. Duodenum

E. Jejunum

F. Kidney

G. Liver

H. Meatus

I. Nephron

J. Pancreas

K. Urethra

L. Saliva

Copyright © 2018 Elsevier Canada, a division of Reed Elsevier Canada, Ltd.

Match the correct pituitary hormone with the effect it has on the body.

76. _____ Growth hormone

77. _____ Thyroid-stimulating hormone (TSH)

78. _____ Adrenocorticotropic hormone (ACTH)

79. _____ Antidiuretic hormone (ADH)

80. _____ Oxytocin

A. Enables thyroid gland function

B. Prevents the kidneys from excreting excessive amounts of water

C. Causes the uterine muscles to contract during childbirth

D. Causes growth of muscles, bones, and other organs

E. Stimulates the adrenal gland

Match the action of the hormone with the correct hormone.

81. _____ Released by pancreas and regulates sugar in blood

82. _____ Sex hormone secreted by testes

83. _____ Sex hormone secreted by ovaries

84. _____ Regulates metabolism

85. _____ Regulates calcium levels in body

86. _____ Stimulates body to produce energy during emergencies

A. Epinephrine

B. Estrogen

C. Insulin

D. Parathyroid hormone

E. Testosterone

F. Thyroxine

Match the special cells or substances in the immune system to their function in protecting the body.

87. _____ Antibodies

88. _____ Antigens

89. _____ Phagocytes

90. _____ Lymphocytes

91. _____ B lymphocytes (B cells)

92. _____ T lymphocytes (T cells)

A. Cause the body to produce antibodies

B. Produce antibodies

C. Cause the production of antibodies that circulate in the plasma

D. Destroy invading cells or attract other cells that destroy invading cells

E. Attack and destroy abnormal or unwanted substances

F. Digest and destroy microorganisms and other unwanted substances

Copyright © 2018 Elsevier Canada, a division of Reed Elsevier Canada, Ltd.

FILL IN THE BLANKS

93. Skeletal muscles are attached to _____ and cause _____ of body parts.

94. What is the function of the nervous system? _____ _____

95. What are the five senses?

    a. _____

    b. _____

    c. _____

    d. _____

    e. _____

96. Three small bones in the middle ear _____ the sound and transmit it to the _____ _____. The small bones in the middle ear are called the _____, _____, and _____ _____.

97. Describe the function of the digestive system. _____ _____

98. The undigested portion of food that passes from the body through the rectum and anus is called ___ _____.

99. Urine is made up of waste products filtered out of the _____.

100. What are the functions of the ovaries?

    a. _____

    b. _____

101. What effects do mineralocorticoid hormones have on the body?

    _____

    _____

    _____

Copyright © 2018 Elsevier Canada, a division of Reed Elsevier Canada, Ltd.

LABELLING

102. Identify the type of joint in each drawing. Name a joint in the body that moves like each one.

A   B

a. _____

b. _____

103. Label the parts of the brain indicated on the drawing.

a. _____

b. _____

c. _____

104. Name the structure and function of the six main parts of the heart indicated on the drawing.

a. _____

_____

b. _____

_____

c. _____

_____

d. _____

_____

e. _____

_____

f. _____

_____

Copyright © 2018 Elsevier Canada, a division of Reed Elsevier Canada, Ltd.

105. Name the structures of the respiratory system indicated on the drawing.

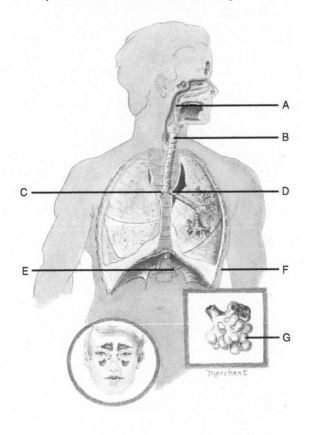

106. Name the structures of the digestive system indicated on the drawing.

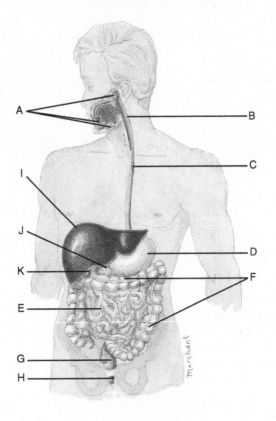

a. _____

b. _____

c. _____

d. _____

e. _____

f. _____

g. _____

a. _____

b. _____

c. _____

d. _____

e. _____

f. _____

g. _____

h. _____

i. _____

j. _____

k. _____

Copyright © 2018 Elsevier Canada, a division of Reed Elsevier Canada, Ltd.

107. Name the structures of the urinary system indicated on the drawing.

108. Name the structures of the parts of the male reproductive system indicated on the drawing.

a. _____

b. _____

c. _____

d. _____

a. _____

b. _____

c. _____

d. _____

e. _____

f. _____

g. _____

h. _____

i. _____

Copyright © 2018 Elsevier Canada, a division of Reed Elsevier Canada, Ltd.

109. Name the structures of the external female genitalia indicated on the drawing.

a. _____

b. _____

c. _____

d. _____

e. _____

f. _____

g. _____

Copyright © 2018 Elsevier Canada, a division of Reed Elsevier Canada, Ltd.

CROSSWORD

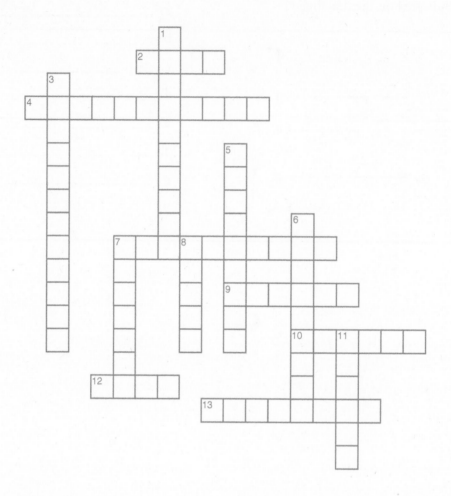

Across

2. Blood vessel that carries blood back to the heart
4. Involuntary muscle contractions in the digestive system that move food through the alimentary canal
7. Substance in red blood cells that carries oxygen and gives blood its colour
9. Blood vessel that carries blood away from the heart
10. Group of cells with the same function
12. Basic unit of body structure
13. Protection against a disease or infection; the person will not get or be affected by the disease

Down

1. Burning of food for heat and energy by the cells
3. Process in which the lining of the uterus breaks up and is discharged from the body through the vagina
5. Tiny blood vessel; food, oxygen, and other substances pass from the capillaries to the cells
6. Process of physically and chemically breaking down food so that it can be absorbed for use by the cells
7. Chemical substance secreted by the glands into the bloodstream
8. Group of tissues with the same function
11. Organs that work together to perform special functions

Copyright © 2018 Elsevier Canada, a division of Reed Elsevier Canada, Ltd.

Growth and Development

TRUE OR FALSE

Circle T for true, or circle F for false.

1. **T F** Three-month-old infants can raise their heads and shoulders when lying on their stomachs.

2. **T F** Toilet training is usually completed by the age of 1 ½ years.

3. **T F** Three-year-olds are able to play with other children.

4. **T F** Young adulthood is the time when partners spend more time alone together.

5. **T F** Adolescents begin to think about careers and what to do after high school graduation.

6. **T F** The term *growth* refers to the physical changes that can be measured and that occur in a steady and organized manner.

7. **T F** Development is a change in psychological and social functioning.

8. **T F** Children should develop at the same rate.

9. **T F** A 4-year-old child has a strong preference for the parent of the same sex.

10. **T F** At 8 years of age, peer-group activities and opinions are important to the child.

11. **T F** Puberty begins when reproductive organs begin to function.

12. **T F** During young adulthood, hobbies and pastimes can be pursued since more free time is available.

Copyright © 2018 Elsevier Canada, a division of Reed Elsevier Canada, Ltd.

MULTIPLE RESPONSE

From the list below, choose all the correct answers.

13. Which of these are among the six basic principles of growth and development?
    A. Growth and development occur from the moment of birth until death.
    B. The process is from simple to complex.
    C. Growth and development occur from head to foot and from the centre of the body outward.
    D. Growth and development occur in a sequence, order, and pattern; each stage lays the foundation for the next stage.
    E. Growth and development occur from the moment of fertilization until death.
    F. Growth and development occur at a set pace.
    G. Each stage of growth and development has its own characteristics and developmental tasks.

MULTIPLE CHOICE

Circle the correct answer.

14. The stage of infancy is the first:
    A. 4 weeks of life
    B. 3 months of life
    C. 6 months of life
    D. Year of life

15. Which reflexes does the infant need for feeding?
    A. The Moro and startle reflexes
    B. The rooting and sucking reflexes
    C. The grasping and Moro reflexes
    D. The rooting and grasping reflexes

16. At what age are solid foods usually introduced to an infant?
    A. Fifth to seventh month
    B. Eighth month
    C. Ninth or tenth month
    D. Eleventh or twelfth month

17. A toddler should be able to:
    A. Use a spoon and cup
    B. Ride a bike
    C. Help set the table
    D. Name parts of the body

18. During which stage do children begin playing with other children?
    A. Infancy
    B. The toddler years
    C. The preschool years
    D. Middle childhood

19. Reproductive organs begin to function and secondary sex characteristics appear during which stage?
    A. Late childhood
    B. Preadolescence
    C. Puberty
    D. Early adulthood

20. Middle adulthood is from about:
    A. 25 to 35 years
    B. 30 to 40 years
    C. 40 to 50 years
    D. 40 to 65 years

21. Middle adulthood is usually a time when:
    A. Families are started
    B. People learn to live with a partner
    C. Children are grown and leave home
    D. People need to prepare for death

22. What stage of growth and development includes the following developmental tasks: a time of rapid growth, and psychological and social maturity?
    A. Late adulthood
    B. Young adulthood
    C. Adolescence
    D. The toddler years

Copyright © 2018 Elsevier Canada, a division of Reed Elsevier Canada, Ltd.

23. What stage of growth and development includes the following developmental tasks: increasing the ability to communicate with and understand others; performing self-care activities; learning the physical differences between the sexes; learning right from wrong and good from bad; learning to play with others; and developing family relationships?
    A. Puberty
    B. Young adulthood
    C. Preschool
    D. Newborn

MATCHING

Match the correct age at which a child is expected to develop each of the following skills.

24. _____ Speaks in short sentences

25. _____ Usually protective of younger brothers and sisters

26. _____ Learn to tell time

27. _____ Smiles and follows objects with the eyes

28. _____ Can eat table food

29. _____ Can hold a rattle

30. _____ Reacts to the word "no"

31. _____ Begins to bite and chew finger foods

32. _____ Plays with the toes

A. 2 months
B. 3 months
C. 5 months
D. 6 months
E. 8 months
F. 1 year
G. 3 years
H. 5 years
I. 7 years

Copyright © 2018 Elsevier Canada, a division of Reed Elsevier Canada, Ltd.

Match the behaviour or physical change with the correct age.

33. _____ Do not like being teased or criticized and are sensitive about how others treat them

34. _____ Temper tantrums and saying "no" are common

35. _____ In girls, pelvis becomes broader, fat appears on hips and chest, and budding of breasts occurs

36. _____ Movements are uncoordinated and lack purpose

37. _____ Select partner and learn to live together; develop intimate relationships

38. _____ May be able to stand when holding on to something

39. _____ Bowel training usually is complete

40. _____ Awkward movements occur because of rapid growth in height and weight

41. _____ Recognize that male and female bodies are different

42. _____ More permanent teeth appear; movements are faster and more graceful

43. _____ Weight control becomes a problem as metabolism and physical activity slow down

44. _____ May cheat to win, but they like rules and try to follow them

45. _____ Baby teeth are lost, and replacement with permanent teeth begins

A. Birth–4 weeks

B. 8 months

C. 2 years

D. 2 ½ years

E. 3 years

F. 5 years

G. 6 years

H. 7 years

I. 8 years

J. 10–14 years

K. Adolescence

L. Young adulthood

M. Middle adulthood

Copyright © 2018 Elsevier Canada, a division of Reed Elsevier Canada, Ltd.

Match the following statements with the correct reflex of an infant.

46. _____ Produced by touching the cheeks

47. _____ When cheek is touched, baby turns head in the direction of touch

48. _____ A loud noise causes infant to throw arms apart and extend legs

49. _____ When palm of hand is touched, baby closes fingers around object

A.   Moro (startle) reflex

B.   Rooting reflex

C.   Sucking reflex

D.   Grasping reflex

Match the developmental task with the correct age group.

50. _____ Accepting the changes in body and appearance

51. _____ Developing leisure-time activities

52. _____ Gaining control of bowel and bladder functions

53. _____ Becoming independent from parents and adults

54. _____ Learning to eat solid foods

55. _____ Developing a conscience and morals

56. _____ Learning to get along with peers

57. _____ Developing a satisfactory sex life

A.   Infancy (birth to 1 year)

B.   Toddler (1 to 3 years)

C.   Preschooler (3 to 6 years)

D.   Middle childhood (6 to 8 years)

E.   Late childhood (9 to 12 years)

F.   Adolescence (12 to 18 years)

G.   Young adulthood (18 to 40 years)

H.   Middle adulthood (40 to 65 years)

Copyright © 2018 Elsevier Canada, a division of Reed Elsevier Canada, Ltd.

Match the developmental task with the correct age group.

58. _____ Developing new friends and keeping friendships with peers

59. _____ Using words to communicate with others

60. _____ Learning to live with a partner

61. _____ Developing a good feeling and attitude about self

62. _____ Developing stable sleep and feeding patterns

63. _____ Performing self-care activities

64. _____ Tend to confide and seek advice from peers

A. Infancy (birth to 1 year)

B. Toddler (1 to 3 years)

C. Preschooler (3 to 6 years)

D. Middle childhood (6 to 8 years)

E. Late childhood (9 to 12 years)

F. Adolescence (12 to 18 years)

G. Young adulthood (18 to 40 years)

FILL IN THE BLANKS

According to your textbook, at what age is a child expected to develop each of the following skills?

65. _____ Child learns to write rather than print

66. _____ Capable of bladder control during the day

67. _____ Knows male and female bodies are different

68. A _____ is a baby in the first 4 weeks after birth.

Copyright © 2018 Elsevier Canada, a division of Reed Elsevier Canada, Ltd.

Caring for Mothers and Infants

TRUE OR FALSE

Circle T for true, or circle F for false.

1. **T** **F** Never leave a baby unattended, or with a sibling, in a tub of water.

2. **T** **F** Formula may be heated safely in a microwave.

3. **T** **F** Extra bottles of formula can be stored in the refrigerator and used within 24 hours.

4. **T** **F** Disposable diapers are changed only when the baby has a bowel movement.

5. **T** **F** All disposable diapers can be flushed down the toilet when soiled.

6. **T** **F** The cord stump dries up and falls off in 7 to 10 days.

7. **T** **F** Cord stump care is given every time a bath is given.

8. **T** **F** The diaper is applied loosely while the circumcision is healing.

9. **T** **F** It is important to respond to the cries of the baby or to feed the baby when he or she is hungry in order to help the baby feel secure and loved.

10. **T** **F** If a baby is "fed on demand," the baby is fed on a regular schedule.

11. **T** **F** To reduce the chance of infection, thoroughly rinse bottles and other equipment in cool water.

12. **T** **F** If the baby has had a large bowel movement or has a rash, the genital area should be washed with cold water.

13. **T** **F** When diapering a boy, the cloth diaper is folded in front. For diapering girls, the diaper is folded in back.

Copyright © 2018 Elsevier Canada, a division of Reed Elsevier Canada, Ltd.

14. **T   F**   It is important to plan well when bathing a baby because once you start, you cannot leave the baby unattended.

15. **T   F**   When you are giving the baby a sponge bath, the head is washed at the end of the bath.

16. **T   F**   It is important to keep babies' nails short to prevent them from scratching themselves.

17. **T   F**   It is best to trim a baby's nails when he or she is awake so the baby is not frightened.

18. **T   F**   The mother will have an abdominal incision if her baby is delivered by Caesarean section.

19. **T   F**   Diarrhea can quickly upset the baby's water balance and harm the baby.

MULTIPLE RESPONSE

From the list below, choose all of the correct answers.

20. When changing a baby on a table or sofa, you can prevent injury by:
    A. Wrapping a belt around the baby and table top to keep the baby secure
    B. Keeping one hand on the baby at all times
    C. Gathering all supplies before beginning the diaper change
    D. Placing a baby monitor nearby and listening for sounds if you must leave the baby unattended

21. Which health reasons or personal beliefs would most likely influence parents to choose to have their son circumcised?
    A. Better hygiene of the genital area
    B. To possibly prevent certain cancers
    C. To prevent the foreskin from getting caught in trouser zippers in the future
    D. Male circumcision is a religious practice of the parents.

22. What signs and symptoms would tell you that an infant may be ill?
    A. Jaundice
    B. Redness or drainage around the cord stump or circumcision
    C. Normal temperature
    D. Limpness and slowness to respond
    E. Occasional screaming or crying
    F. Flushed or pale skin
    G. Heavy perspiration
    H. Rash
    I. Soft, rhythmic respirations
    J. Coughing or sneezing
    K. Reddened or irritated eyes
    L. Turning head to one side or putting a hand to one ear (signs of an ear infection)
    M. Very hungry; eating
    N. Vomiting most of the feeding or between feedings
    O. Soft stools
    P. Stiff neck
    Q. Signs of dehydration (i.e., fewer than six wet diapers a day, dark yellow urine, decreased saliva and tears, dry lips, dry and wrinkled skin, sunken eyes and top of head)
    R. Frequent watery, green, mucusy, or foul-smelling stools

23. What ways would be helpful to assist a mother with breastfeeding?
    A. Wash your hands and remind the mother to wash hers
    B. Tell the mother to assume a comfortable position
    C. Change the baby's diaper if necessary Bring the baby to the mother
    D. Tell the mother to cover the baby and herself with a blanket
    E. Help the mother burp the baby
    F. Change the baby's diaper after the feeding if necessary
    G. Lay the baby in the mother's bed if the baby is asleep
    H. Record what time the baby nursed and how long on each side, and report any problems or concerns

Copyright © 2018 Elsevier Canada, a division of Reed Elsevier Canada, Ltd.

24. To what types of baby formula must you add water?
    A. Ready-to-feed formula
    B. Powdered formula
    C. Concentrated formula

25. What measures are important to follow for bottle-feeding a baby?
    A. Place the bottle in the microwave to warm up the formula.
    B. Tilt the bottle to check the flow of formula dripping out of the nipple.
    C. Assume a comfortable position for feeding.
    D. Hold the baby close to you.
    E. Tilt the bottle so that the neck of the bottle and the nipple are always filled.
    F. Lay the baby down comfortably and prop up the bottle for the feeding.
    G. Burp the baby after about half the formula and at the end of the feeding.
    H. Keep feeding the baby until all the formula is finished.
    I. Place remaining formula in the refrigerator.
    J. Wash the bottle, cap, and nipple after the feeding.

26. What are good methods for burping a baby?
    A. Hold the baby over your shoulder and gently pat or rub the baby's back.
    B. Support the baby in a sitting position on your lap. Gently pat or rub the baby's back.
    C. If the baby is under 3 months, bounce the baby gently.

27. Cord care includes:
    A. Keeping the cord moist at all times
    B. Washing your hands before and after contact with the umbilical area
    C. Keeping the cord clean by gently wiping around the base of the cord with a clean cloth moistened with warm water
    D. Keeping the top of the diaper below the cord
    E. Reporting any signs of infection (e.g., redness, odour, drainage from the cord)

28. What safety measures should be followed when bathing a baby?
    A. Never leave the baby alone on a table or in the bathtub.
    B. Hold the baby securely throughout the bath.
    C. Keep room temperature between 18 and 20°C.
    D. Water temperature must be between 37.8 and 40.6°C. Measure bath temperature with a thermometer or test with the inside of your wrist.

29. Signs and symptoms of postpartum complications include:
    A. Fever of 38°C or higher
    B. Chills, poor appetite, fatigue, nausea, or vomiting
    C. Lochia that soaks a sanitary pad within 1 hour of application
    D. Foul-smelling lochia
    E. Large number of clots in the lochia
    F. Painful, burning, or difficult urination
    G. Mild abdominal or perineal pain
    H. Bleeding, redness, swelling, or drainage from a Caesarean-section incision
    I. Leg pain, tenderness, or swelling
    J. Breast pain, warmth, tenderness, or swelling
    K. Feelings of severe depression

MULTIPLE CHOICE

Circle the correct answer.

30. Which of these statements is true about cloth diapers?
    A. When soiled, they are placed in the garbage.
    B. They can be easily composted.
    C. They are cheaper to use than disposable diapers.
    D. Cloth diapers are never washed in hot water.

Copyright © 2018 Elsevier Canada, a division of Reed Elsevier Canada, Ltd.

31. How do you remove formula from bottle nipples?
    A. Place them in the sterilizer
    B. Squeeze hot, soapy water through the nipples
    C. Clean them with a bottle brush
    D. Wash them with cool, clean water

32. Which of the following concerns should the mother discuss immediately with her doctor or nurse practitioner?
    A. The baby "spits up" during burping.
    B. The baby's bowel movement consists of hard, formed stool.
    C. The baby's cord stump is dry.
    D. The baby stops crying when she is picked up and cuddled.

33. A sign of infection in the cord stump would be:
    A. A dried, blackened piece of tissue
    B. Redness or odour at the site
    C. Slight bleeding when the stump falls off
    D. Softening around the base of the cord

34. When a baby boy is circumcised, which of the following is true?
    A. The penis will look red, swollen, and sore.
    B. Urination will be difficult until it is healed.
    C. The area will completely heal in 4 to 6 days.
    D. Circumcision results in shortening the length of the penis.

35. When the area of the circumcision is cleaned, what is applied to prevent the penis from sticking to the diaper?
    A. Alcohol
    B. Soap and water
    C. Powder
    D. Petroleum jelly

36. What part of the body is cleaned with cotton swabs during a sponge bath?
    A. Nostrils
    B. Eyes
    C. Ears
    D. No part of the body

37. Which of the following indicates a vaginal or uterine infection in a postpartum woman?
    A. Dark red discharge 3 to 4 days after delivery
    B. An increase in lochia flow with activity
    C. A foul-smelling lochia
    D. Lochia alba that continues for 2 to 6 weeks after delivery

FILL IN THE BLANKS

38. Explain how you would prepare each of the following forms of baby formula:

    a. Ready-to-feed formula _____

    _____

    b. Powdered formula _____

    _____

    c. Concentrated formula _____

    _____

39. What should you do if a baby has diarrhea?

    _____

    Why? _____

    _____

Copyright © 2018 Elsevier Canada, a division of Reed Elsevier Canada, Ltd.

Caring for the Young

TRUE OR FALSE

Circle T for true, or circle F for false.

1. **T**   **F**   Do not tie pacifiers or other items around a baby's neck.

2. **T**   **F**   Television during mealtime relaxes the child and stimulates appetite.

3. **T**   **F**   It is not your duty to provide a stable, secure, or safe atmosphere for the family.

4. **T**   **F**   You should try to develop positive relationships with all family members.

5. **T**   **F**   You should punish the misbehaving child the way the parents would.

6. **T**   **F**   Bedtime rituals should be eliminated if the child is ill.

7. **T**   **F**   It is dangerous to leave any child unsupervised in the home.

8. **T**   **F**   Touching the child to provide comfort should depend on the child's culture.

MULTIPLE RESPONSE

From the list below, choose all of the correct answers.

9. Which of the statements below are true for preventing injuries in infants and children?
   A. Use baby walkers only outside.
   B. Keep the highchair away from stoves, tables, and counters.
   C. Secure the child into a highchair using the waist and crotch straps.
   D. Do not use a baby walker.
   E. Check children in cribs once a night.
   F. Make sure there are no toys or soft, fluffy items in the crib.
   G. Ensure the crib mattress is soft and bendable.
   H. Avoid using safety plugs in electrical outlets.
   I. Do not let electrical cords hang down from tables or counters.
   J. Do not let children wear necklaces, strings, cords, or other items around their necks.
   K. Hang items with strings, cords, or elastic only around cribs or playpens.
   L. Keep all poisonous substances in a high, locked area away from children.
   M. Do not store harmful substances in food containers or juice bottles.
   N. Keep childproof caps on harmful substances.

Copyright © 2018 Elsevier Canada, a division of Reed Elsevier Canada, Ltd.

10. Ways to prevent children from drowning in or around the home include:
  A. Teaching children how to swim at a young age if they play near swimming pools unattended
  B. Keeping bathroom doors closed to prevent drowning in toilets or bathtubs
  C. Keeping diaper pails locked
  D. Keeping sinks, tubs, basins, and buckets empty when not in use

11. What safety measures can prevent burns in children?
  A. Do not drink cold liquids around children.
  B. Make sure children are not around hot utensils, irons, or dishes from the oven.
  C. Heat a baby bottle only in the microwave.
  D. Always shake the contents of a baby bottle thoroughly before giving it to the baby.
  E. Test the temperature of food and fluids before you give them to the baby.
  F. Always test bath water using your hand.
  G. Do not let a child touch faucet handles.
  H. Keep pot handles facing inward on the stove, away from a child's reach.
  I. Do not let children cook at the stove.
  J. Do not let children near curling irons or electric curlers.
  K. Do not let electric cords from irons, coffee pots, toasters, and so on hang down where a child can reach them.
  L. Do not let children play around ovens, fireplaces, or other heat sources.
  M. Supervise a child lighting firecrackers.
  N. Do not let a child play unsupervised outdoors if there are open firepits or burning leaves in the yard.

12. What measures can help to prevent poisoning in children?
  A. Keep all harmful substances in high, locked areas where children cannot reach them.
  B. Keep cigarette butts away from a child's reach.
  C. Store all harmful substances in their original containers.
  D. Never store harmful materials or liquids in food or juice containers.
  E. Never store harmful materials near foods.
  F. Never mix cleaning products, as mixing them could produce harmful fumes.
  G. Never call medications or vitamins "candy."
  H. Do not leave your purse or work bag sitting out where children can reach it, especially if it contains medications or harmful substances.
  I. Keep plants away from toddlers and infants.
  J. Do not let children play near walls with chipped paint; the paint may contain lead.
  K. Keep phone numbers for the Poison Control Centre, police, and ambulance handy near the phone.

Copyright © 2018 Elsevier Canada, a division of Reed Elsevier Canada, Ltd.

MULTIPLE CHOICE

Circle the correct answer.

13. How can you prevent choking injuries?
    A. Use rolled towels to prop up bottles while baby is feeding.
    B. Never give infants and young children foods such as hot dogs, peanuts, or popcorn.
    C. Always use strings or cords to secure a child's hood and waistline.
    D. Position infants on their stomachs for sleep.

14. Children are vaccinated to _____ certain contagious infections.
    A. Prevent them from developing (catching)
    B. Cure them of
    C. Reduce the symptoms of
    D. Infect them with

15. Which of the following statements about vaccinating children is true?
    A. If vaccinations were to be discontinued, the rate of disease would go down.
    B. Children need to be vaccinated against viral meningitis.
    C. Vaccines can be given to infants only.
    D. Vaccinations prevent the spread of a certain variety of pathogens.

16. As a general rule, children should stay home from school or day care if:
    A. They drink normally but pick at their food
    B. They have a temperature of 37.5°C (99.5°F) and sleep soundly at night
    C. They have a temperature over 38°C (100.4°F), diarrhea, and vomiting
    D. They have been on antibiotics for 36 hours

17. Reye's syndrome is:
    A. A rare congenital condition caused by nuclear radiation
    B. A rare but often fatal illness linked to taking aspirin to treat influenza or chicken pox
    C. A condition caused by an allergy to acetaminophen (Tylenol)
    D. A common congenital condition caused by a mother drinking alcohol while pregnant

18. One of the five most common reasons children stay home from school or day care is that they:
    A. Do not wish to go to school
    B. Ate too many hot dogs at a birthday party
    C. Have test anxiety
    D. Have conjunctivitis

19. One of the main principles in supporting challenging children is to:
    A. Sternly punish bad behaviours
    B. Encourage and reinforce good behaviours
    C. Yell at them to let them know who is the boss
    D. Never give in to their demands

20. Which of the following statements about vaccination is true?
    A. Vaccination can cause autism.
    B. The risk of not being vaccinated is greater than any risk from vaccination.
    C. In the case of an outbreak, no child can be prevented from attending class.
    D. There is no legislation in Canada that requires a child to be vaccinated.

Copyright © 2018 Elsevier Canada, a division of Reed Elsevier Canada, Ltd.

MATCHING

Match the safety measure used with the correct risk factor.

21. _____ Never store cleaning products in easy-to-reach areas.

22. _____ Measure the temperature of bath water.

23. _____ Keep one hand on a child lying on a table if you must look away.

24. _____ Do not prop up a baby bottle with a rolled-up towel or blanket.

25. _____ Teach children not to eat unknown foods, leaves, stems, seeds, berries, nuts, or bark.

26. _____ Never leave children unattended in a bathtub.

27. _____ Keep cords for drapes, blinds, and shades out of reach of children.

28. _____ Make sure there is nothing in the crib that the baby can stand on (like large stuffed toys or firm bumper pads).

A. Burns

B. Suffocation

C. Falls

D. Poisoning

FILL IN THE BLANKS

29. Children are at special risk for suffocation. What safety measures can be used to prevent suffocation in infants and children?

a. _____

b. _____

c. _____

d. _____

e. _____

f. _____

g. _____

h. _____

i. _____

j. _____

Copyright © 2018 Elsevier Canada, a division of Reed Elsevier Canada, Ltd.

Caring for Older Adults

TRUE OR FALSE

Circle T if the statement promotes a client's rights, and circle F if it does not.

1. **T   F**   Encourage the client to wear a hospital gown at all times.

2. **T   F**   Protect the client's right to privacy.

3. **T   F**   Encourage the client to get counselling if the client's sexual attitudes are different from yours.

4. **T   F**   Knock before you enter a room.

5. **T   F**   Older clients have the right to be sexual.

6. **T   F**   Discourage single older clients from developing new relationships.

7. **T   F**   Couples in a long-term care facility should be allowed to share the same room.

8. **T   F**   Same-sex couples should not be allowed to share a room.

9. **T   F**   Separation from children can cause loneliness in an older client.

10. **T   F**   Men usually live longer than women.

11. **T   F**   Clients who do not speak English have a greater risk of suffering from loneliness and isolation.

12. **T   F**   The skin of an older adult is fragile and easily injured.

13. **T   F**   The older adult may have decreased mobility, which would decrease the risk of falls.

14. **T   F**   Activity and diet can slow the loss of bone and muscle strength.

15. **T   F**   Decreased kidney function may cause the urine to be more concentrated.

16. **T   F**   Men may have difficulty urinating because of prostate gland enlargement.

17. **T   F**   The support worker can help the client at risk for urinary tract infections by providing extra fluids.

Copyright © 2018 Elsevier Canada, a division of Reed Elsevier Canada, Ltd.

MULTIPLE RESPONSE

From the list below, choose all of the correct answers.

18. How can the support worker facilitate breathing in the older client?
    A. Avoid the use of heavy bed linens over the client's chest.
    B. Turn and reposition the client at least every 4 hours.
    C. Encourage deep breathing.
    D. If the client is on bed rest, keep the head of the bed flat.
    E. Encourage activity.

19. What are some ways in which older adults may express closeness and intimacy without having intercourse?
    A. Holding hands
    B. Touching
    C. Caressing
    D. Embracing

MULTIPLE CHOICE

Circle the correct answer.

20. Which of these statements about sexuality for older adults is true?
    A. Love, affection, and intimacy are an important part of life at any age.
    B. Older adults are unable to masturbate.
    C. It is not normal for older adults to be sexual.
    D. A decline in the female hormone estrogen increases sexual desire.

21. Which of these statements is true about sexuality and the older adult?
    A. After menopause, women are no longer interested in having sexual relations.
    B. A man cannot have an erection when he gets older.
    C. Sexual relationships are psychologically and physically important to the older adult.
    D. Orgasm may be less intense and longer in duration than in younger adults.

22. Which of the following physical changes is most likely to cause confusion or behavioural changes in an older client?
    A. Respiratory infections
    B. Lack of exercise
    C. Reduced blood flow to the brain
    D. Poor fluid intake

23. Which of the following is true in regard to depression in older adults?
    A. Depression is an inevitable part of the aging process.
    B. Older adults are more likely to report their depression than younger adults.
    C. Depression in older adults may go unrecognized.
    D. Depression in older adults must be treated with medication.

24. Why should older adults avoid using heating pads?
    A. Their skin has overactive oil glands and may burn easily.
    B. They will not be able to manage the heating controls.
    C. Heating pads can impair circulation.
    D. Decreased sensitivity to heat may increase the risk of burns.

25. Older adults often complain that food has no taste. This happens because:
    A. Memory is shorter in older adults.
    B. The number of taste buds decreases with age.
    C. The ability to feel heat and cold decreases.
    D. A progressive loss of brain cells occurs.

Copyright © 2018 Elsevier Canada, a division of Reed Elsevier Canada, Ltd.

MATCHING

Match the statement about physical changes in the older person with the body system affected.

26. _____ Decrease in bone strength

27. _____ Change in sleeping patterns

28. _____ Less blood flows through narrowed arteries

29. _____ Folds, lines, and wrinkles appear

30. _____ Lung tissue becomes less elastic

31. _____ Decreased appetite

32. _____ Urine becomes concentrated

A. Integumentary

B. Musculo-skeletal

C. Nervous

D. Cardiovascular

E. Respiratory

F. Digestive

G. Urinary

Match the body system to the correct care measures described.

33. _____ Performing range-of-motion exercises

34. _____ Providing a sweater and a lap blanket for a client who is cold

35. _____ Allowing the older client to rest or nap more during the day

36. _____ Placing the client in a semi-Fowler's position

A. Integumentary

B. Nervous

C. Musculo-skeletal

D. Respiratory

FILL IN THE BLANKS

Indicate whether the examples given are:
A. *A benefit of working*
B. *A benefit of retirement*
C. *A negative aspect of retirement*

37. _____ Time to travel

38. _____ More leisure time

39. _____ Poor health and aging

40. _____ Increased medical bills with less income

41. _____ Personal fulfillment and usefulness

42. _____ Friendships formed with coworkers

43. _____ Reduced income forces lifestyle changes

44. _____ Time to do as you wish

45. _____ Meeting basic needs of love, belonging, and self-esteem

46. _____ Reward for a lifetime of work

Copyright © 2018 Elsevier Canada, a division of Reed Elsevier Canada, Ltd.

Indicate whether each of the effects of aging listed is:
A. **Physical**
B. **Psychological**
C. **Social**

47. _____ Greying hair

48. _____ Preparing for one's own death

49. _____ Death of a partner

50. _____ Slower movements

51. _____ Retirement

52. What are two common causes of loneliness in older clients?

    a. _____

    b. _____

53. What happens to the roles of children and parents as the parent ages?

    _____

54. What are some ways loneliness in older people can be prevented?

    a. _____

    b. _____

    c. _____

55. Why are there usually more widows than widowers?

    _____

56. When a partner dies, how is the other partner affected?

    a. Serious _____ and _____ problems may occur.

    b. May lose _____ or attempt _____.

57. In Canada, older clients who do not speak English or French often have greater loneliness and isolation than others. What are some of the reasons for this?

    a. Relatives and friends who share cultural values may _____.

    b. Clients may not have anyone _____ and may not

    _____.

Copyright © 2018 Elsevier Canada, a division of Reed Elsevier Canada, Ltd.

58. How do these physical changes affect the safety of older adults?

    a. Skin is fragile and easily injured _____

    b. Fewer nerve endings _____

    c. Decreasing strength and muscle atrophy _____

    d. Bones become brittle _____

    e. Reduced sense of touch and pain _____

    f. Reduced blood flow to brain; loss of brain cells _____

59. Older clients often complain of feeling cold. What are some ways you can safely provide warmth?

    a. _____

    b. _____

    c. _____

60. How can loss of bone and muscle strength be slowed?

    a. _____

    b. _____

61. Touch and sensitivity to _____ and _____ are reduced with aging.

62. Urine may be more concentrated because of _____ and _____.

63. Urinary frequency or urgency may occur because _____ weaken and _____ decreases.

64. Why should you make sure an older adult reduces fluid intake after 5 p.m.?

    _____

Copyright © 2018 Elsevier Canada, a division of Reed Elsevier Canada, Ltd.

Safety

TRUE OR FALSE

Circle T for true, or circle F for false.

1. **T F** An electrical plug not being grounded may cause a fire.

2. **T F** Visitors need to be reminded not to smoke in a room with supplemental oxygen, even if the facility has a "No Smoking" policy.

3. **T F** To prevent sparks, you must turn off electrical equipment before unplugging it.

4. **T F** You should attempt to put out a fire before sounding a fire alarm.

5. **T F** All fire extinguishers are effective for any fire.

6. **T F** Disinfectants and cleaning solutions are hazardous substances.

7. **T F** Warnings, words, pictures, and symbols on hazardous substances may be removed after opening the container.

8. **T F** Check the material safety data sheet (MSDS) after cleaning up a leak or spill or disposing of a hazardous substance.

9. **T F** When using restraints, the most restrictive device is used.

10. **T F** Apply a restraint only after receiving instructions about its proper use.

11. **T F** Always follow manufacturers' instructions when using restraints.

12. **T F** Sheets, towels, or other items can be used to position and stabilize a client on the toilet.

MULTIPLE RESPONSE

From the list below, choose all of the correct answers.

13. What physical changes in some older adults place them at risk for accidents?
    A. Stiff joints and weakened muscle groups
    B. Improved balance and coordination
    C. Increased sensitivity to heat, smell, taste, and touch
    D. Diminished vision and hearing
    E. Memory problems

Copyright © 2018 Elsevier Canada, a division of Reed Elsevier Canada, Ltd.

14. Why should you avoid calling a client by name as a method of identifying the client?
    A. Some clients may be confused and unaware of their name.
    B. Some clients who are disoriented may answer to any name.
    C. Some clients with hearing difficulties may not hear you correctly.

15. The support worker can prevent falls when giving care by:
    A. Taping cords and wires near the wall and away from the path for walking
    B. Using high-gloss floor wax to prevent tripping
    C. Cleaning up water and other spills immediately
    D. Keeping lights on low dimmers to decrease glare
    E. Reporting frayed, torn, or bumpy rugs and carpets
    F. Rearranging the client's furniture to a better arrangement
    G. Using nonslip rubber bath mats or nonslip strips in bathtubs and showers
    H. Making sure that the client's footwear and clothing fit properly
    I. Ensuring the client's shoes and slippers are nonskid

16. Injury prevention measures include:
    A. Encouraging the client to wear reading glasses when up and about
    B. Ensuring crutches, canes, and walkers have nonskid tips
    C. Checking the client carefully and often, especially a client with risk factors
    D. Using pillows, wedge pads, or seats to position the client as the care plan directs
    E. Keeping wheelchair wheels unlocked when stationary

17. Under the occupational health and safety (OH&S) legislation, what must your employer do to ensure your safety?
    A. Have written safety policies
    B. Train and educate employees about these safety policies
    C. Create a health and safety committee to identify workplace hazards and investigate accidents
    D. Respond to reports of workplace hazards
    E. Warn employees about safety hazards and correcting these hazards whenever possible
    F. Make sure that all necessary equipment is available and in good working order

18. OH&S legislation states the employee's responsibilities are:
    A. Follow all safety policies and procedures
    B. Use all recommended protective equipment and clothing
    C. Decide which concerns should be addressed to the supervisor or the health and safety committee
    D. Complete an incident report after an accident in the specified time

19. Safety measures aimed at preventing burns include:
    A. Telling clients about the dangers of wearing tight-fitting clothing while cooking
    B. Keeping clients who smoke a designated distance away from the doors of the facility
    C. Following safety guidelines and the care plan when applying heat and cold
    D. Testing the temperature of food by dipping a clean spoon into the food and touching the inner aspect of your lower arm with it
    E. Testing the water in the tub, shower, or basin with your hand before bathing an adult or helping an adult bathe
    F. Checking for "hot spots" in the bath water, and mix the water well by moving your hand back and forth in it
    G. Relying on the client to check the temperature of the bathwater before bathing
    H. Allowing the client to eat or drink food that is only warm and not hot

Copyright © 2018 Elsevier Canada, a division of Reed Elsevier Canada, Ltd.

20. Incident reports are used by employers and health and safety committees to:
    A. Identify recurring problems
    B. Determine who is following health and safety policies
    C. Determine which steps were followed after the injury or incident occurred
    D. Justify cost-saving measures

21. What safety information should the support worker know and use when handling hazardous substances?
    A. How to safely handle the product
    B. The cost of the product
    C. How to safely use the product
    D. How to safely freeze the product
    E. First aid measures required in case of an accident or emergency
    F. Instructions for disposing of the product

22. Call bells:
    A. Can be ignored if the client is known to call needlessly
    B. Should always be placed within the client's reach on her strong or dominant side
    C. Enable the client to call for assistance
    D. Can be removed from a client's bedside if the staff are frequently alerted

23. What information about hazardous materials can be found on the Workplace Hazardous Materials Information System (WHMIS) label?
    A. Risk phrases that describe the health hazard
    B. Supplier information
    C. Hazard symbol
    D. Cost of the product
    E. Precautionary statements that describe safety measures to take when using the product
    F. First aid measures in case of accident or emergency
    G. Reference to the material safety data sheet (MSDS)

24. Restraints may be used only:
    A. When absolutely necessary
    B. When the client is in imminent danger of harming others
    C. When a client is refusing to eat
    D. When a client actively threatens to harm himself
    E. As a last resort and after less-restrictive measures have failed

25. Which of the following statements are true in regard to restraints?
    A. A restraint is any device that restricts or limits movement.
    B. Support workers are responsible for determining who should have a restraint applied.
    C. Restraints can cause emotional harm and physical injury.
    D. Unnecessary restraint is false imprisonment.
    E. Restraints are used to discipline certain clients.

26. What alternatives to restraints can be used by a support worker when giving care?
    A. Use diversions, such as TV or music, to calm and distract the client.
    B. Avoid following routines and habits since they obviously do not work.
    C. Provide attention and companionship.
    D. Turn up the volume of the TV or radio so the client will hear it.
    E. Avoid explaining procedures and care measures to reduce confusion.
    F. Closely supervise the client.
    G. Allow the client to wander in a safe area.
    H. Promote uninterrupted sleep.
    I. Meet food, fluid, and elimination needs promptly.
    J. If ordered, help the client use padded hip protectors, pillows, wedge cushions, and posture and positioning aids.
    K. Follow safety precautions to prevent falls; if ordered, use floor cushions and roll guards.
    L. Take away call bells, as they are a safety hazard.

Copyright © 2018 Elsevier Canada, a division of Reed Elsevier Canada, Ltd.

27. How can you meet a restrained client's psychological needs?
    A. Treat the person with kindness, caring, respect, and dignity.
    B. Toilet the client every 6 hours.
    C. Visit the person often.
    D. Offer repeated explanations and reassurance.
    E. Be a good listener.

28. What information should be reported to the nurse when you are caring for a restrained client?
    A. The type of restraint applied
    B. The reason for the restraint
    C. Safety measures taken, as listed in the care plan, such as whether bed rails are padded or raised
    D. The time the restraint was applied
    E. The time the restraint was removed
    F. The care given when the restraint was removed
    G. Skin colour and condition
    H. The pulse felt in the restrained part
    I. Complaints of a tight restraint; difficulty breathing; and pain, numbness, or tingling in the restrained part

MULTIPLE CHOICE

Circle the response that correctly completes the sentence.

29. A chemical restraint is a _____ used to control behaviour or movement.
    A. Belt
    B. Jacket
    C. Food
    D. Medication

30. Which of the following statements about restraint use is true?
    A. Most facilities have limited policies about the use of restraints.
    B. Restraints cannot be used without prior informed consent given.
    C. A wheelchair belt is not considered to be a restraint.
    D. Items such as bedsheets can be used to restrain a client.

31. When a client is restrained, the support worker must check the client at least every _____.
    A. 5 minutes
    B. 15 minutes
    C. Hour
    D. 2 hours

32. Which of these statements is correct regarding restraints?
    A. Certain drugs may be a form of restraint.
    B. Restraints may be used for staff convenience.
    C. Restraints are never used to protect a client from harming himself or herself or others.
    D. The staff determines who should be restrained.

33. Restraints that are too big or loose can increase the risk for _____.
    A. Cuts
    B. Bruises
    C. Strangulation
    D. Suffocation

34. When a client's clothing is on fire, you should _____ the client and cover him or her with a _____ or coat to smother the flames.
    A. Roll, blanket
    B. Hug, curtain
    C. Hug, blanket
    D. Roll, curtain

35. It is important to exercise personal safety measures at all times to avoid injury. If visiting a client in the home, one safety precaution would be to:
    A. Position yourself in the corner of the room
    B. Remove shoes or boots and throw them at the client if the client is being abusive
    C. Try to reason with the client or family member who is abusive or making sexual demands
    D. Be cautious in hallways, elevators, and stairwells

Copyright © 2018 Elsevier Canada, a division of Reed Elsevier Canada, Ltd.

36. Which is a good personal safety measure to take when driving to and from work?
    A. Always use a seat belt.
    B. Never park near people; choose remote, empty areas.
    C. Do not take your keys out until you are at your car.
    D. Never carry cash with you at any time.

37. If someone tries to force you into a vehicle, you should:
    A. Cry softly
    B. Push your thumbs into the attacker's eyes
    C. Avoid resisting and go into the vehicle
    D. Crouch in a fetal position

38. Accident risk factors include:
    A. Natural disasters
    B. Impaired vision and hearing
    C. Suffocation
    D. Sleeping

39. Which of the following sets of factors puts a client at increased risk for falls?
    A. Confusion, disorientation, and memory problems
    B. Increased joint mobility and muscle strength
    C. Visual impairment, strange surroundings, and improved reaction time
    D. Regular exercise and diet habits, proper use of medications

40. In a facility, falls are most likely to occur:
    A. During shift changes
    B. During meal times
    C. When visitors are present
    D. While care is being given

41. Which factor increases a client's risk of falling?
    A. Awareness of surroundings
    B. A history of falls
    C. Well-fitting footwear
    D. Muscle coordination

42. A client who has balance problems is:
    A. At risk for memory problems
    B. Suffering from impaired hearing
    C. At risk of falling
    D. Taking medication

43. Which of the following can help to prevent falls?
    A. Spills on the floor
    B. Scatter rugs
    C. Night lights
    D. Clutter

44. A person has a chair alarm. Which is true?
    A. It serves the same purpose as a night light.
    B. You need to respond immediately to the alarm.
    C. Alarms are used only at night.
    D. Alarms reduce the need to watch the client.

45. Bed rails are padded to:
    A. Prevent the person from getting caught between the rails and the mattress
    B. Provide privacy for the person
    C. Prevent the person from climbing out of bed
    D. Decrease agitation

46. What should you do if you find that a smoke detector does not work in a home where you are giving care?
    A. Replace the battery.
    B. Call the fire department.
    C. Notify the nurse and the family.
    D. This is not your responsibility; do not get involved.

47. If a fire occurs, which of these steps should be done first?
    A. Use a fire extinguisher to put out the fire.
    B. Close all doors and windows.
    C. Announce "Fire" in a loud voice.
    D. Move people who are in danger to a safe place.

Copyright © 2018 Elsevier Canada, a division of Reed Elsevier Canada, Ltd.

48. Suffocation can occur because:
A. A person chokes on a piece of food
B. A person is given a tub bath
C. Restraints are applied correctly
D. Dentures fit properly

49. When an accident or error occurs, it is correct to:
A. Report the accident or error immediately to your supervisor
B. Report the incident only if a client is injured
C. Call the family immediately
D. Call the doctor or ambulance

50. If your car breaks down, a good safety practice would be to:
A. Stay in the car and call police if you have a cellphone
B. Ask for a ride to a police station if someone stops to help
C. Walk to the nearest place where you can get help
D. Get out of the car and try to flag down a ride for help

51. If you feel uncomfortable or threatened in a home setting, you should first:
A. Speak to the person who is threatening you
B. Go to a safe place immediately and call your supervisor
C. Resign from your job
D. Call a co-worker to come to the home to assist you

52. Which of the following would be a threat to your safety in home care?
A. Denial of meal breaks, drinking water, or bathroom use
B. Inadequate heat or ventilation
C. Being subject to name-calling or obscene language
D. All of the above

MATCHING

Match the description or example with the correct restraint.

53. _____ A drug is given that is not required to treat the client's medical symptoms.

54. _____ An attached tray keeps the client from getting up.

55. _____ Hands are covered to prevent the client from removing the dressing.

A. Chemical restraint
B. Mitt restraint
C. Geriatric chair

Match the safety measure used with the correct risk factor.

56. _____ Measure the temperature of bath water.

57. _____ Keep the client's room free of clutter.

58. _____ Open doors and windows if you notice gas odours.

59. _____ Store cleaners, medicines, and hazardous substances in the original containers.

A. Burns
B. Suffocation
C. Falls
D. Poisoning

Copyright © 2018 Elsevier Canada, a division of Reed Elsevier Canada, Ltd.

Match the safety measure used with the correct risk factor.

60. _____ Do not allow smoking in bed.

61. _____ Do not prop up a baby bottle with a rolled-up towel or blanket.

62. _____ Use nonslip strips on the floor next to the bed and in the bathroom.

A. Burns

B. Suffocation

C. Falls

Match the accident risk factor with the possible outcome or injury.

63. _____ Can harm herself or others because she cannot understand what is happening

64. _____ May take wrong medication or dosage or poison himself because cannot read labels

65. _____ Has problems smelling smoke or gas, so is unaware of fire

66. _____ Cannot hear fire alarms or sirens, so cannot move to safety

67. _____ Has not learned the difference between safety and danger, so is unaware of hazardous situations

68. _____ May be aware of danger but is unable to move to safety

A. Impaired awareness of surroundings

B. Impaired vision

C. Impaired hearing

D. Altered sense of smell or touch

E. Paralysis

F. Developmental stage or age

Match the accident risk factor with the possible outcome or injury.

69. _____ Injury resulting from being unaware that certain people, places, or things may be safety hazards

70. _____ Movements slower and less steady; balance affected

71. _____ Can trip on toys, rugs, furniture, electrical cords

72. _____ Easily burned because of problems sensing heat and cold

73. _____ Cannot hear explanation or instructions, so may take wrong medication or dosage

74. _____ May develop pressure sores from lack of movement

75. _____ Unaware that mixing these without proper guidance can cause illness or death

A. Impaired awareness of surroundings

B. Impaired vision

C. Impaired hearing

D. Altered sense of touch

E. Paralysis

F. Medications

G. Developmental stage or age

Copyright © 2018 Elsevier Canada, a division of Reed Elsevier Canada, Ltd.

FILL IN THE BLANKS

76. Where would you find information about a hazardous substance found in the workplace?

    _____

77. What are some behaviours that would allow for the use of restraints?

    a. _____

    b. _____

    c. _____

78. If the support worker applies a restraint unnecessarily, he or she could face _____

    _____.

79. The client or substitute decision maker must give _____ for the use of

    restraints. The support worker _____ (can or cannot) provide the information about

    restraints and obtain the signed consent.

80. When a person is restrained, the support worker must make sure basic needs are met by doing the

    following:

    a. The person must be checked at least_____.

    b. Meet the person's needs for _____, _____,

       _____, and _____.

81. Several staff members may be needed to apply restraints because _____

    _____.

82. Why can confusion increase when a person is restrained?

    _____ or

    _____.

83. When applying restraints, the person should be positioned in _____, and

    any bony areas and skin should be _____ to prevent

    _____ and _____.

84. Restraints that are too small cause _____, _____

    _____, or _____.

85. What personal safety measures can you take to reduce your risk for assaults?

    a. _____
    b. _____
    c. _____
    d. _____
    e. _____
    f. _____

86. How can you use your car keys as a weapon?

    _____
    _____

87. How can you use your body as a weapon if you are attacked?

    a. _____
    b. _____
    c. _____

LABELLING

88. What are two safety problems with the plug in the figure?

    a. _____
    b. _____

Copyright © 2018 Elsevier Canada, a division of Reed Elsevier Canada, Ltd.

Preventing Infection

TRUE OR FALSE

Circle T for true, or circle F for false.

1. **T F** Microbes cannot survive in reservoirs.

2. **T F** Microbes are destroyed by a warm, dark environment.

3. **T F** Items can be sterilized in the home with boiling water.

4. **T F** If you must transport a client with an infection that requires droplet or airborne precautions out of his or her room, the client must wear a disposable gown.

5. **T F** When you remove gloves, the inside is considered clean.

6. **T F** If a sterile item touches a clean item, the sterile item is contaminated.

7. **T F** If a clean item touches a sterile item, the clean item is contaminated.

8. **T F** If a sterile item is above your waist, it is contaminated.

9. **T F** Microbes exist in six different forms.

10. **T F** Animals are common reservoirs for microbes.

11. **T F** The environment must be warm and bright for microbes to survive.

12. **T F** Hands should be held up throughout the handwashing procedure.

13. **T F** Paper towels are used to turn off hand-operated water faucets to avoid contaminating the hands.

14. **T F** Mr. Fox has an infection caused by a wound on his leg. This infection can exit Mr. Fox's body through his wound.

15. **T F** Pathogens from Mr. Fox's infection cannot enter another person's body through a portal of entry.

16. **T F** Portals of entry can include mucous membranes.

17. **T F** The easiest and most important way to prevent the spread of infection is by eating well and staying fit.

18. **T F** A gown is contaminated when wet and should be removed.

19. **T F** Nosocomial or health care–associated infections (HAIs) are acquired after a person's release from a health care facility.

20. **T F** The respiratory tract is one of the most common sites for nosocomial or health care–associated infections (HAIs).

21. **T F** When cleaning equipment, the support worker should rinse the item in cold water first.

22. **T F** Chemical disinfectants are used to clean reusable items.

23. **T F** An effective and cheap disinfectant for home use may be made by mixing 1 cup of bleach with 3 cups of water.

24. **T F** After preparing the effective and cheap disinfectant solution from question #23, it should be labelled "toxic cleaner."

25. **T F** A simple way to sterilize items in the home is to pour boiling water over them.

26. **T F** If an item is sitting on the floor, it is considered to be contaminated.

27. **T F** When you are finished using a sharp object (such as a razor), after giving care, you should place it in the garbage.

28. **T F** After a mask has been worn, the outside part is considered to be contaminated.

29. **T F** Gloves should be changed between tasks (procedures) on the same client.

30. **T F** When you enter the room of a client with contact precautions, you should never wear gloves.

MULTIPLE RESPONSE

From the list below, choose all of the correct answers.

31. Signs and symptoms of a systemic infection include:
    A. Behavioural changes (especially in older adults)
    B. Swelling and redness of the area
    C. Presence of dandruff and itchy scalp
    D. Low body temperature
    E. Chills
    F. Decreased pulse
    G. Increased respiratory rate
    H. Fatigue and loss of energy
    I. Increased appetite
    J. Discharge from the infected area that may have a foul odour

32. Nancy is a support worker caring for a client in the home. She should wash her hands:
    A. Approximately one half hour before and after giving care
    B. Only when the hands are visibly soiled
    C. After contact with her own or another's blood, body fluids, secretions, or excretions
    D. After touching objects that are contaminated (e.g., soiled linens, garbage bags)
    E. Before and after preparing and handling only foods that must be heated
    F. Before feeding the client
    G. While wearing gloves
    H. After personal body functions (e.g., going to the bathroom, sneezing)

Copyright © 2018 Elsevier Canada, a division of Reed Elsevier Canada, Ltd.

33. What guidelines should be followed when cleaning equipment?
    A. Wear personal protective equipment (PPE) when cleaning items that may be contaminated with blood, body fluids, secretions, or excretions.
    B. Wash the item with soap and bleach.
    C. Scrub the item thoroughly.
    D. After cleaning, rinse the item in cold water.
    E. Dry the item.

34. Standard Practices are guidelines used to prevent the spread of infection from:
    A. Blood
    B. Only people who live high-risk lifestyles
    C. All body fluids, secretions, and excretions
    D. All hair and skin products
    E. Nonintact skin (skin with open breaks)
    F. Mucous membranes

35. You should allow a client to see your face before you put on personal protective equipment:
    A. Because children may be afraid if they cannot see your face
    B. Because clients with confusion or dementia may be afraid if they cannot see your face
    C. To avoid clients thinking you are there to rob them

36. Aseptic measures the support worker can use in the health care facility to control the transmission of infection include:
    A. Assisting clients with handwashing as necessary
    B. Washing hands properly morning, afternoon, and evening
    C. Cleaning, disinfecting, and sterilizing equipment, as appropriate
    D. Maintaining personal hygiene
    E. Keeping vaccinations up to date
    F. Keeping tables, countertops, wheelchair trays, and other surfaces clean and dry
    G. Washing contaminated areas with tap water
    H. Providing for the client's skin care and oral hygiene, according to the care plan
    I. Covering nose and mouth with a mask when coughing or sneezing
    J. Ensuring clients have their own care equipment, and not sharing items among clients
    K. Taking equipment and supplies from one client's room and using with another client to reduce expenses
    L. Holding equipment and linens close to the body
    M. Covering bedpans and commodes with a lid when transporting
    N. Avoiding sitting on a client's bed
    O. Not using items that have touched the floor for 5 seconds or more
    P. Disinfecting tubs, showers, shower chairs, bedpans, urinals, and commodes after each use

37. When you are assigned to care for a client in isolation, you should tell the nurse if you have:
    A. Tattoos under your uniform
    B. Broken skin on your face, arms, or legs
    C. Fever
    D. Vomiting
    E. Diarrhea
    F. Sore throat
    G. Asthma

Copyright © 2018 Elsevier Canada, a division of Reed Elsevier Canada, Ltd.

38. Types of sharps containers that may be used in home care include:
    A. Containers according to employer policy
    B. Containers that you can easily open to empty
    C. Containers that are puncture-resistant
    D. Containers that are leak-proof

39. When you care for a client with an infection, what precautions should be used when handling contaminated laundry?
    A. Sort or rinse linen only in client care area.
    B. Hold soiled linens away from your uniform. Wear gloves.
    C. Remove soiled linens by folding them with the cleanest areas in the centre.
    D. Linen contaminated with blood, body fluids, secretions, or excretions must be placed in a sturdy, leak-proof laundry bag labelled with the biohazard symbol.
    E. Bag soiled linen in the room where it was used.

MULTIPLE CHOICE

Circle the correct answer.

40. When your hands are contaminated while working in a health care facility, you should wash them for at least:
    A. 3 to 5 minutes
    B. 2 minutes
    C. 15 to 20 seconds
    D. 1 minute

41. Which of these statements reflects the use of proper aseptic technique?
    A. Take clean, unused equipment from one person's room to another room.
    B. Clean from the dirtiest area to the cleanest area.
    C. Wear personal protective equipment as needed.
    D. Keep tables and other surfaces clean by wiping them down with the client's facecloth.

42. Here is a list of common aseptic practices that you should use. Which one is the most important for preventing the spread of infection?
    A. Bathing, washing hair, and brushing teeth regularly
    B. Washing cooking utensils with soap and water
    C. Covering nose and mouth when coughing or sneezing
    D. Washing hands immediately before and after client care as necessary

43. Transmission-Based Precautions are used:
    A. When caring for all clients
    B. When caring for clients with open wounds
    C. Depending on how the pathogen is spread
    D. Only when caring for clients with a respiratory infection

44. When you are caring for a client who is in isolation, what should you do if you drop clean linens on the floor?
    A. Pick them up and return them to the stack of clean linens.
    B. They are contaminated and should be thrown in the trash.
    C. They are contaminated and should be placed in the dirty linen container.
    D. Use them immediately so they are mixed with clean linens.

45. Paper towels are used in isolation:
    A. To handle contaminated items
    B. Under clean items or objects
    C. To turn faucets on and off
    D. For all of the above

46. Standard Practices should be used:
    A. Only when you think a person has an infection
    B. Only when you are changing soiled linens
    C. Only when you have open skin wounds
    D. When caring for all persons at all times

Copyright © 2018 Elsevier Canada, a division of Reed Elsevier Canada, Ltd.

47. When you are removing gloves after giving care, which part is considered "clean"?
    A. The inside
    B. The outside
    C. Both sides
    D. Neither side

48. When transporting a client who is in isolation, the client should wear a mask:
    A. At all times
    B. Until he or she reaches the destination
    C. If he or she is on airborne or droplet precautions
    D. Only while in an elevator

49. Which of the following aseptic measures will control the portal of entry?
    A. Make sure all clients have their own personal care equipment.
    B. Make sure drainage tubes are correctly connected.
    C. Cover your nose and mouth when coughing or sneezing.
    D. Keep drainage containers below drainage sites.

50. If a container is labelled "biohazard," it contains materials that are:
    A. Sterile
    B. Radioactive
    C. Contaminated
    D. Poisonous

51. Which, if any, of these gloves can be reused after cleaning?
    A. Sterile gloves
    B. Disposable gloves
    C. Utility gloves
    D. None of the above

52. Which of the following statements about wearing gloves is correct?
    A. Remove and discard torn or punctured gloves immediately.
    B. Wear the same gloves when giving care to both people in a semi-private room.
    C. Practise hand hygiene while wearing your gloves.
    D. Hand hygiene is not necessary if you wear gloves.

53. When is double-bagging of biohazardous waste necessary?
    A. Any time contaminated items are removed from the client's room
    B. When the client has contact precautions
    C. When materials are contaminated with body fluids
    D. When the outside of the biohazard bag has been contaminated

54. When putting on sterile gloves, which of the following steps is correct?
    A. Lift the second glove by touching only the inside of the glove.
    B. Pick up the second glove by reaching under the cuff with your hand.
    C. Hold the thumb of your first gloved hand away from your second hand as you put on the glove.
    D. Place the glove package below waist height.

55. How can you help to prevent a client's decrease in self-esteem when the client is in isolation?
    A. Discourage visits by family and friends
    B. Maintain distance between you and the client
    C. Arrange to spend time to visit with the client
    D. Remain in the room only for a short time

Copyright © 2018 Elsevier Canada, a division of Reed Elsevier Canada, Ltd.

FILL IN THE BLANK

56. What do the following statements describe? _____
    • They exist in five different forms.
    • They can live in a person, a plant, an animal, soil, food, water, or other material.
    • They need water, nourishment, and oxygen to live.
    • They all need a warm, dark environment to live and may be destroyed by heat and light.

58. The environment must be _____ and _____
    for microbes to survive. They also need _____to live.

59. Why do you hold your hands down throughout the handwashing procedure?
    _____

60. Why do you turn off the water by using a paper towel to touch the hand-operated faucets?
    _____

61. What is the easiest and most important way to prevent the spread of a person's infection?
    _____.

62. The most common sites for nosocomial or health care–associated infections (HAIs) are
    a. _____
    b. _____
    c. _____
    d. _____

63. Utility or rubber household gloves should be worn when using a chemical disinfectant because it can
    _____.

64. When using Standard Practices, masks, eye protection, and face shields are worn during
    _____.

65. What are some of the rules to follow when caring for a client under Transmission-Based Precautions?

a. _____

b. _____

c. _____

d. _____

e. _____

DIAGRAMS

66. Identify the parts of the hands that are frequently missed during handwashing by shading them in with a pencil in the image below.

67. Identify the part of the gown that is considered contaminated after use by shading in the contaminated area with a pencil in the image below.

A   B

Copyright © 2018 Elsevier Canada, a division of Reed Elsevier Canada, Ltd.

68. Identify the part of the sterile field (shown below) that is considered contaminated by shading in the area with a pencil in the image below.

Copyright © 2018 Elsevier Canada, a division of Reed Elsevier Canada, Ltd.

Skin Care and Prevention of Wounds

TRUE OR FALSE

Circle T for true, or circle F for false.

1. T F When giving a back massage, massage the bony areas thoroughly.

2. T F Clients sitting in a chair should be reminded to shift their weight every hour.

3. T F When bathing or drying the client, rub vigorously.

4. T F To prevent pressure ulcers, you must frequently check clients who are incontinent to ensure they are not lying on wet linens.

5. T F When applied, adhesive tape should circle the entire body part to prevent swelling.

6. T F Make sure you collect all equipment needed before you begin to change a nonsterile dressing.

7. T F When changing a dressing, you should make sure that the client looks at his or her wound.

8. T F When changing a dressing, you need to wear gloves only if there is drainage.

9. T F You should never apply lotion to a skin crease.

10. T F A stasis ulcer is caused by poor blood return through the veins.

11. T F A skin tear is a very deep cut in the skin.

12. T F Skin tears commonly occur in the head and chest.

13. T F When oxygen and nutrients get into the cells, skin, and tissues, pressure ulcers will occur.

14. T F When a client slides down in a bed or chair, shearing occurs. Blood vessels and tissues are damaged.

Copyright © 2018 Elsevier Canada, a division of Reed Elsevier Canada, Ltd.

15. **T** **F** In obese clients, pressure ulcers can develop where skin surfaces press against each other, causing a decrease in blood flow.

16. **T** **F** Heel protectors reduce pressure on the heels by lowering them.

17. **T** **F** A flotation pad or cushion is placed in a pillowcase so the pad does not touch the skin.

18. **T** **F** You should check with the nurse before using soap on a client who is at risk for pressure ulcers because soap can moisturize the skin.

19. **T** **F** Skin should be kept clean and dry and free of moisture from urine, stool, perspiration, and wound drainage.

20. **T** **F** When very small amounts of drainage are expected, a drain is applied to enable the drainage to leave the wound.

21. **T** **F** Scabs and scars are complications of wound healing that are surgical emergencies.

MULTIPLE RESPONSE

From the list below, choose all of the correct answers.

22. Strategies for preventing skin tears include:
    A. Keeping the skin dry and avoiding all moisturizers or skin softeners
    B. Offering fluids
    C. Dressing and undressing the client carefully
    D. Dressing the client in soft clothing with long sleeves and long pants
    E. Keeping your fingernails short and smoothly filed
    F. Keeping the client's fingernails short and smoothly filed
    G. Not wearing rings with raised or large stones
    H. Following safety guidelines when lifting and transferring clients
    I. Preventing friction and shearing during lifting, moving, transferring, and repositioning (e.g., using a transfer sheet or pad)
    J. Avoiding the use of pillows to support arms and legs
    K. Being patient and calm when the client resists care
    L. Padding bed rails and wheelchair arms, footrests, and leg supports
    M. Providing good lighting to help prevent the client from bumping into furniture or walls

23. What are common causes of skin breakdown and pressure ulcers?
    A. Pressure
    B. Age
    C. Friction
    D. Shearing

Copyright © 2018 Elsevier Canada, a division of Reed Elsevier Canada, Ltd.

24. You can prevent shearing and friction by:
    A. Using proper lifting, positioning, and transferring procedures
    B. Applying a thin layer of powder to the bottom sheets
    C. Never raising the head of the bed more than 30 degrees
    D. Use a turning pad (or sheet) to move and turn the client in bed.

25. Clients at risk for pressure ulcers are those who:
    A. Are confined to a bed or chair
    B. Require moderate to complete help in moving
    C. Have loss of bowel or bladder control
    D. Have fair to good nutrition
    E. Have altered mental awareness
    F. Have problems sensing pain or pressure
    G. Have circulatory problems
    H. Are younger
    I. Are obese or very thin

26. Why are pillows and blankets used to prevent pressure ulcers?
    A. To prevent skin from being in contact with skin
    B. To reduce moisture and friction between skin surfaces
    C. To keep the client well hydrated

27. Signs that a pressure ulcer is beginning and that therefore should be reported include:
    A. Shivering and a drop in body temperature
    B. An increase in blood pressure
    C. Pale skin
    D. A warm, reddened area

28. Common sites for stasis ulcers are:
    A. Lower legs
    B. Upper arms
    C. Feet
    D. Face and neck

29. What are the risk factors for the development of arterial ulcers?
    A. High blood pressure
    B. Diabetes
    C. Poor diet
    D. Aging
    E. Smoking
    F. Osteoporosis

30. When observing a wound's appearance, what should you continue to monitor?
    A. If the wound is red and swollen
    B. If the area around the wound is warm to the touch
    C. If sutures, staples, or clips are intact or broken
    D. If wound edges are closed or separated, or if the wound has broken open
    E. If the client has complained of the wound getting itchy at times.

31. What are the functions of wound dressings?
    A. They protect wounds from injury and microbes.
    B. They absorb drainage.
    C. They remove dead tissue.
    D. They promote comfort.
    E. They keep the wound warm.
    F. They cover unsightly wounds.
    G. They provide a moist environment for wound healing.
    H. When bleeding is a problem, pressure dressings help control bleeding.

32. How should tape be applied to secure a dressing?
    A. Apply tape to the top, middle, and bottom of the dressing.
    B. Extend the tape several centimetres beyond each side of the dressing.
    C. Place one piece of adhesive tape across the middle of the dressing.

33. What types of tape do not cause allergic reactions?
    A. Paper tape
    B. Plastic tape
    C. Cloth tape

Copyright © 2018 Elsevier Canada, a division of Reed Elsevier Canada, Ltd.

34. If a client has a draining wound, you can help improve the client's appetite by:
    A. Covering the wound with an airtight dressing
    B. Using room deodorizers as directed
    C. Keeping drainage containers out of the client's sight
    D. Offering foods that are strongly scented to mask any odour of wound drainage
    E. Removing soiled dressings promptly from the room

35. How should you remove tape and old dressings from a wound?
    A. Hold the skin down and gently pull the tape toward the wound. Remove adhesive from the skin.
    B. Lift the dressing very gently, and keep the soiled side of the dressing out of the client's sight.
    C. Pull the dressing off as quickly as you can.

36. You can assist a client with a wound by:
    A. Allowing pain medications to take effect before giving care
    B. Ensuring the client stays on complete bed rest until the wound is fully healed
    C. Carefully observing the wound and reporting any signs or symptoms of infection immediately
    D. Implementing Standard Practices during all client care

MULTIPLE CHOICE

Circle the correct answer.

37. Which of the following is a cause of skin breakdown?
    A. Good nutrition and hydration
    B. Decreased mobility
    C. Increased circulation
    D. A regular exercise program

38. Which of the following practices are intended to prevent skin tears in clients?
    A. Taking daily baths
    B. Keeping your fingernails short and smoothly filed
    C. Wearing jewellery with large stones
    D. Wearing a clean uniform daily

39. To prevent pressure ulcers, the health care team may place the client on a surface such as:
    A. A firm mattress
    B. A foam, air, alternating air, or gel mattress
    C. Plastic or rubber material
    D. A bed board

40. Which of the following measures is helpful in preventing pressure ulcers?
    A. Position the client at a 45 degree angle.
    B. Reposition the client every 6 hours.
    C. Massage around bony and reddened areas.
    D. Keep the client's heels on the bed.

41. Which of the following measures would help to prevent stasis ulcers?
    A. Making sure the client's clothing fits tightly
    B. Having the client wear elastic stockings as ordered by the doctor
    C. Massaging any reddened area over pressure points
    D. Having the client trim his own toenails weekly

42. Why may pain medication be given before a dressing change?
    A. To reduce discomfort during the dressing change
    B. To prevent the client from looking at the wound
    C. To prevent the client from seeing your nonverbal responses
    D. To prevent contamination of the wound

Copyright © 2018 Elsevier Canada, a division of Reed Elsevier Canada, Ltd.

43. When you are removing an old dressing, it should be:
    A. Shown to the client
    B. Removed quickly from the wound with a quick pull
    C. Removed so that the soiled side is turned away from the client's sight
    D. Placed in the client's garbage can

44. Movement and ambulation can contribute to wound healing by:
    A. Ensuring the wound dressing stays in place
    B. Keeping the client's skin clean and dry
    C. Encouraging better oxygenation of tissue cells
    D. Preventing discoloration of the wound scar

45. Which practice is intended to prevent pressure sores in the client's coccyx area?
    A. Never trimming the client's toenails if the client has diabetes
    B. Brushing the client's teeth, flossing gently, and inspecting the mouth for food particles
    C. Washing bony prominences with gentle soap, rinsing, and drying well.
    D. Encouraging deep breathing and helping the client to cough up phlegm.

46. Clients who are in pain are at greater risk for developing pressure sores because:
    A. They may be more likely to eat and drink well
    B. They cry more and require more emotional support
    C. They are less likely to require pain medication
    D. They are less likely to move and reposition themselves

47. Clients with infected and draining wounds will require more of which two nutrients?
    A. Calcium and iron
    B. Protein and vitamin C
    C. Potassium and phosphorus
    D. Vitamins A and D

Copyright © 2018 Elsevier Canada, a division of Reed Elsevier Canada, Ltd.

MATCHING

Match the type of wound with the correct description.

48. _____ Wound containing large amounts of bacteria

49. _____ Wound that does not heal easily

50. _____ Wound created for therapy

51. _____ Wound resulting from trauma

52. _____ Wound occurring from surgical entry of the urinary, reproductive, respiratory, or gastro-intestinal system

53. _____ Wound that is not infected; microbes have not entered wound

54. _____ Wound in which dermis, epidermis, and subcutaneous tissue are penetrated; muscle and bone may be involved

55. _____ Wound with high risk of infection

56. _____ Wound in which tissues are injured, but the skin is not broken

57. _____ Wound in which skin or mucous membrane is broken

58. _____ Wound in which dermis and epidermis of the skin are broken

A. Persistent wound

B. Clean wound

C. Clean-contaminated wound

D. Closed wound

E. Contaminated wound

F. Dirty (infected) wound

G. Full-thickness wound

H. Intentional wound

I. Open wound

J. Partial-thickness wound

K. Unintentional wound

Match the type of wound drainage with the correct description.

59. _____ Thin, watery drainage that is blood tinged

60. _____ Thick green, yellow, or brown drainage

61. _____ Bloody drainage

62. _____ Clear, watery fluid

A. Purulent drainage

B. Sanguineous drainage

C. Serosanguineous drainage

D. Serous drainage

Match the stage of a pressure ulcer with the correct description.

63. _____ The skin is gone, and underlying tissues are exposed.

64. _____ The skin cracks, blisters, and peels.

65. _____ Drainage is likely.

66. _____ The colour does not return to the skin when pressure is relieved.

A. Stage 1

B. Stage 2

C. Stage 3

D. Stage 4

Copyright © 2018 Elsevier Canada, a division of Reed Elsevier Canada, Ltd.

Match the stage of a pressure ulcer with the correct description.

67. _____ Muscle and bone are exposed and damaged.   A.   Stage 1

68. _____ The skin is red.   B.   Stage 2

69. _____ There may be a shallow crater.   C.   Stage 3

70. _____ The exposed tissue is damaged.   D.   Stage 4

Match the phase of wound healing with the correct statement.

71. _____ Tissue cells multiply to repair the wound.   A.   Inflammatory phase

72. _____ The scar eventually becomes thin and pale.   B.   Proliferative phase

73. _____ Blood supply to the wound increases.   C.   Maturation phase

FILL IN THE BLANKS

74. What is the purpose of heel elevators?

    _____

75. What is the purpose of a drain placed in a wound?

    _____

76. Why should you be careful to control nonverbal communication when changing a dressing?

    _____

77. How can you assist a person with a wound with the following concerns?
    a. Pain and discomfort

    _____

    b. Nutrition

    _____

    c. Infection

    _____

Copyright © 2018 Elsevier Canada, a division of Reed Elsevier Canada, Ltd.

LABELLING

78. Place an X on six areas where pressure ulcers may form on a person lying in the lateral position.

79. Place an X on six areas where pressure ulcers may form on a person lying in the prone position.

80. Place an X on three areas where pressure ulcers may form on a person lying in the Fowler's position.

81. Place an X on four areas where pressure ulcers may form on a person in the sitting position.

Copyright © 2018 Elsevier Canada, a division of Reed Elsevier Canada, Ltd.

82. Identify the stages of pressure ulcers by writing the letter beside each stage number in the correct order. Describe the tissue damage in each one.

Courtesy Laurel Wiersma-Bryant, RN, MSN, Clinical Nurse Specialist, Barnes-Jewish Hospital, St. Louis

    a. Stage _____

    _____

    b. Stage _____

    _____

    c. Stage _____

    _____

    d. Stage _____

    _____

Copyright © 2018 Elsevier Canada, a division of Reed Elsevier Canada, Ltd.

CROSSWORD PUZZLE

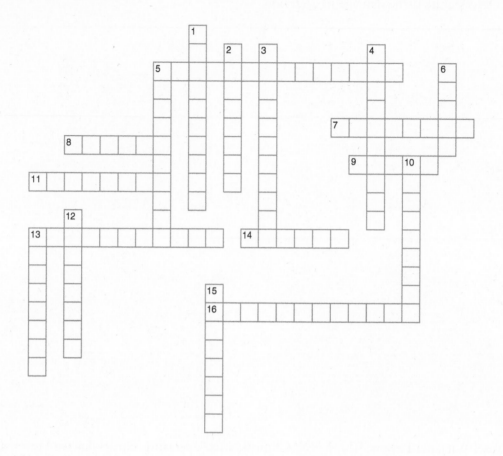

Across

5. Pressure ulcer, pressure sore, bedsore *(2 words)*

7. Thick green, yellow, or brown discharge

8. Clear, watery drainage

9. Condition that results when there is not enough blood supply to organs and tissues

11. Condition in which there is death of tissue

13. Thin, blood-tinged, watery drainage

14. Accident or violent act that injures the skin, mucous membranes, bones, and internal organs

16. Separation of wound along with protrusion of abdominal organs

Down

1. Open wound with torn tissues and jagged edges

2. Partial-thickness wound caused by scraping away or rubbing of the skin

3. Open wound caused by poor blood return to the heart from the legs and feet *(2 words)*

4. Excessive loss of blood in a short period of time

5. Separation of wound layers

6. Break in the skin or mucous membranes

10. Closed wound caused by blow to the body

12. Open wound with clean, straight edges; usually intentionally produced with a sharp instrument

13. Break or rip in skin that separates the epidermis from the underlying tissues *(2 words)*

15. Collection of blood under the skin and tissues

Copyright © 2018 Elsevier Canada, a division of Reed Elsevier Canada, Ltd.

Body Mechanics: Moving, Positioning, Transferring, and Lifting the Client

TRUE OR FALSE

Circle T for true, or circle F for false.

1. **T** **F** Log-rolling keeps the spine straight.

2. **T** **F** When you lift, move, or carry objects, hold them with your arms extended.

3. **T** **F** When lifting an object from the floor, bend from the waist.

4. **T** **F** By using two or more people to help a heavy, weak, or very old client move up in bed, you protect only the client from injury.

5. **T** **F** In some agencies, a turning pad can be an incontinence pad or a folded sheet.

6. **T** **F** When transferring a client to a chair, choose a chair based primarily on how comfortable the chair will be.

7. **T** **F** A client lying in bed or sitting in a chair should be repositioned every 3 to 4 hours.

8. **T** **F** Rubbing of one surface against another is called *friction*.

9. **T** **F** The way in which body parts are aligned with one another is called *base of support*.

10. **T** **F** The skin sticking to a surface, causing the muscles to slide in the direction the body is moving, is called *skinning*.

11. **T** **F** Another name for a transfer or safety belt is a *gait belt*.

12. T F Turning the client as a unit in alignment in one motion is called *body mechanics.*

13. T F Another name for the back-lying or dorsal recumbent position is the *supine position.*

14. T F Another name for the side-lying position is the *sideline position.*

15. T F The semi-sitting position, with the head of the bed elevated 45 to 60 degrees, is called the *Franklin position.*

16. T F A left-side-lying position in which the upper leg is sharply flexed is called the *Sims' position.*

17. T F Another word for *posture* is *body mechanics.*

18. T F A turning sheet or pad is also called a *transfer sheet* or *pad.*

19. T F Sitting on the edge of the bed is called *edging.*

20. T F The position in which the client is placed on his abdomen with his head turned to one side is called the *drone position.*

21. T F A chair used to move clients from one place to another is called a *wheelchair.*

22. T F You can provide a better base of support for lifting by standing with your legs and feet apart for a wide base of support.

23. T F Providing a good base of support will help to reduce the risk of injury.

24. T F When you move a client up in bed, it is important to protect the skin from shaving.

25. T F You should place the pillow against the headboard when moving a client up in bed to prevent her head from hitting the headboard.

26. T F The level of the bed should be raised horizontally when the client is being repositioned to reduce the amount of work the support worker has to do.

27. T F Two staff members work together when raising an older client's head and shoulders to provide more support, for clients with fragile bones and joints.

28. T F A transfer pad is used to keep the bedding neater and to reduce wrinkling.

29. T F A transfer belt is used on men who have poorly fitting trousers to keep them from falling down.

30. T F The seat of the wheelchair is padded to promote the client's comfort.

31. T F Mechanical lifts are used when a client cannot assist with a transfer.

32. T F The number of staff members needed to transfer a client from the bed to a chair or wheelchair depends on the client's physical abilities and condition.

33. T F The *Sims' position* is the right-side-lying position.

34. T F The *supine position* is a back-lying position.

35. T F The *prone position* is difficult for ill clients to maintain.

Copyright © 2018 Elsevier Canada, a division of Reed Elsevier Canada, Ltd.

36. **T**   **F**   When in the supine position, ankles should be elevated on two pillows.

37. **T**   **F**   The *stroke position* is also known as the lateral position.

38. **T**   **F**   To correctly lift an object from the floor, you should use muscles in your shoulders, upper arms, hips, and thighs.

MULTIPLE RESPONSE

From the list below, choose all of the correct answers.

39. When working together, two co-workers can ensure they move the client at the same time by:
     A. One person communicating directions when lifting
     B. Counting to 10
     C. Lifting together

40. It is important for a support worker to follow the guidelines for good body mechanics. These guidelines are:
     A. Assess the situation before you begin lifting
     B. Face your work area
     C. Bend your back and squat when lifting
     D. Tighten your stomach muscles and tuck in your pelvis as you lift
     E. Hold objects close to your body when lifting, moving, or carrying them
     F. Avoid unnecessary bending and reaching
     G. Turn your whole body in sections when changing the direction of your movement

41. How can you provide comfort and safety to a client being lifted or moved in bed?
     A. Check with your supervisor and the care plan about limits or restrictions in moving or positioning that client
     B. While you are moving the client, decide how to move the client and how much help you need
     C. Ask for help before starting the move
     D. Communicate directions with your helper by counting 1–2–3 and then moving together
     E. Move the client in one large movement
     F. Cover and screen the client for privacy
     G. Make sure tubes or drainage containers connected to the client are not pulled, tangled, or pinched during the move
     H. Position the client in good alignment after the move
     I. Make sure linens are wrinkle-free after moving the client

42. Log-rolling is used to turn:
     A. Clients with arthritic spines or knees
     B. Clients recovering from hip fractures
     C. Clients with spinal cord injuries
     D. Clients with facial injuries
     E. Clients recovering from spinal cord surgery

43. What observations should you make when the client is dangling the legs?
     A. Pulse and respirations (if instructed to do so)
     B. The length of time the person's legs dangled
     C. Complaints of dizziness, light-headedness, or difficulty breathing
     D. How well the activity was tolerated
     E. The amount of assistance that you wish you had

44. Before using a lift, make sure:
     A. The client has read the lift policy for your agency
     B. You are trained to use the lift
     C. The lift works
     D. The client's weight does not exceed the lift's weight limit

Copyright © 2018 Elsevier Canada, a division of Reed Elsevier Canada, Ltd.

45. When you position a client, you should follow these safety regulations:
    A. Check with the care plan for the best position for the client.
    B. Ask the client when you should reposition her.
    C. Use good body mechanics.
    D. Ask for help before beginning the process.
    E. Explain the procedure to the client after performing the procedure.
    F. Be gentle when moving the client.
    G. Provide for privacy.
    H. Leave the client in good body alignment.
    I. Use pillows as directed in the care plan for comfort and support.
    J. Make sure linens are wrinkle-free by tucking the top sheet under the mattress.
    K. In facilities, place the call bell within the client's reach.

46. What are the benefits of repositioning a client frequently?
    A. Promotes comfort and well-being
    B. Makes breathing easier
    C. Keeps linens cleaner and fresher smelling
    D. Helps prevent many complications (e.g., pressure ulcers and contractures)

MULTIPLE CHOICE

Circle the correct answer.

47. A transfer sheet or pad is used by placing it under the client:
    A. From the head to above the knees
    B. From the shoulders to the hips
    C. From the head to the hips
    D. From the shoulders to the knees

48. Why should shoes with nonskid soles be worn by the client being transferred to a chair or wheelchair?
    A. To provide a good base of support
    B. To make the client more steady on his feet
    C. To prevent the client sliding or slipping on the floor
    D. To provide strength on the client's weak side

49. When transferring a client to a stretcher:
    A. The client is moved by moving the head first
    B. A transfer belt is used to lift the client
    C. The head of the bed is raised before the transfer
    D. Three or more staff members are needed

50. Body alignment is:
    A. The way the head, trunk, and legs are aligned with each other
    B. The same as *body mechanics*
    C. The base of support
    D. The area on which an object rests

51. Mr. John Dunlop is turned as a unit, with one motion. This is called:
    A. Body mechanics
    B. Log-rolling
    C. Ergonomics
    D. The safety roll

52. Mrs. Renee Nadeau has slid down in bed. Her skin sticks to the bed while her muscles move down. This is called:
    A. Friction
    B. Abrasion
    C. Tension
    D. Shearing

53. When you are giving bedside care, the bed should be:
    A. At its lowest horizontal level
    B. At its highest horizontal level
    C. Level with your waist
    D. In Fowler's position

54. You need to move a client up in bed. To reduce your risk of injury:
    A. Use a transfer belt
    B. Raise the head of the bed prior to moving the client
    C. Instruct the client to place both hands around your neck and shoulders
    D. Get assistance from a co-worker

Copyright © 2018 Elsevier Canada, a division of Reed Elsevier Canada, Ltd.

55. To prevent falls during transfers, you should ensure that wheelchair or shower chair wheels are:
    A. Fully inflated
    B. Locked and aligned correctly
    C. Removed
    D. Positioned sideways and at right angles to the chair

56. Mrs. Arja Gupta has weakness on her left side. Where should you position the wheelchair?
    A. At the foot of the bed
    B. At the head of the bed
    C. Next to the bed on her left side
    D. Next to the bed on her right side

57. When you have to move, turn, or transfer a client, it is always best to:
    A. Use a transfer belt
    B. Have a co-worker help you
    C. Follow the care plan
    D. Use a mechanical lift

58. Before moving, turning, transferring, or lifting a client, you should always:
    A. Explain what you are going to do in a way the client understands
    B. Ask a co-worker to help you
    C. Apply a transfer belt
    D. Use a mechanical lift

59. A no-lift policy means:
    A. You should not bend over to pick up something that fell to the floor
    B. Mechanical lifts need to be used for lifting clients
    C. Only the special lift team is allowed to lift clients
    D. Clients are not allowed to be lifted at any time

FILL IN THE BLANKS

60. The position in which the client is placed on his abdomen with his head turned to one side is called the _____ _____ position.

61. How can you make sure that you and a co-worker both move the person at the same time when working together? _____ _____; _____ _____ _____

62. When a lift sheet is used, _____ _____ and _____ _____ are reduced, and the person can be _____.

63. Why should you move a person to the side of the bed before turning?

64. Why do you pad the seat of the wheelchair?

65. When are mechanical lifts used? _____

Copyright © 2018 Elsevier Canada, a division of Reed Elsevier Canada, Ltd.

FILL IN THE BLANKS

Complete each statement, referring to the illustrations below.

66. The illustration below shows the _____ _____ position.

67. The illustration below shows the _____ _____ position.

68. The illustration below shows the _____ _____ position, with a pillow placed under the _____ _____ to prevent pressure on the toes.

69. The illustration below shows the _____ _____ position, with the feet positioned over _____ _____ _____ _____.

70. The illustration below shows the _____ _____ position.

71. When lifting correctly as in the images below, which muscle groups are used? _____ _____

Copyright © 2018 Elsevier Canada, a division of Reed Elsevier Canada, Ltd.

Exercise and Activity

TRUE OR FALSE

Circle T for true, or circle F for false.

1. **T F** Exercise every joint on every client.

2. **T F** Support the extremity being exercised.

3. **T F** Exercise the joint to the point of pain.

4. **T F** The client should wear soft slippers or sandals when using crutches.

5. **T F** Loose clothing can hang forward and block the client's view of the feet and crutches.

6. **T F** A pouch attached to a walker will always interfere with the client's ability to ambulate.

7. **T F** When a client is on bed rest, some ADLs are allowed, such as feeding and oral hygiene.

8. **T F** Strict bed rest means everything is done for the client.

9. **T F** Bed rest with commode privileges means the client can use the bathroom for elimination needs.

10. **T F** Plantar flexion and footdrop can be prevented by using a footboard.

11. **T F** A trochanter roll can be used to prevent external rotation of the hips and legs.

12. **T F** A hip abduction wedge keeps the hips together.

13. **T F** If a client is falling, you should try to stop the fall.

14. **T F** When ambulating, the cane is used on the strong side.

15. **T F** A walker gives more support than a cane.

MULTIPLE RESPONSE

From the list below, choose all of the correct answers.

16. Which of the following are benefits of bed rest?
    A. Reduces physical activity
    B. Reduces pain
    C. Reduces pressure ulcers
    D. Encourages rest
    E. Promotes healing

17. Which of the following is correct when a client is using a cane?
    A. The cane is used on the weak side.
    B. The client should move the cane forward 15–25 cm at a time.
    C. The client should move the strong leg forward first.

MULTIPLE CHOICE

Circle the correct answer.

18. Which of the following statements correctly describes a type of bed rest?
    A. The client remains in bed but is allowed to perform some activities of daily living (ADLs).
    B. The client can use the bedside commode for elimination needs.
    C. Everything is done for the client; no ADLs are allowed.
    D. All of the above describe bed rest.

19. Which of the following steps would be used to prevent orthostatic hypotension?
    A. Assist the client to lie on the edge of the bed.
    B. Ask the client about weakness, dizziness, or spots before the eyes.
    C. Have the client stand up quickly when getting out of bed.
    D. Measure blood pressure, pulse, and respirations each time the client changes position.

20. Which of the following is a complication of bed rest?
    A. Urinary retention
    B. Diarrhea
    C. Blood clots
    D. Diabetes

21. What is one type of range-of-motion exercises that a support worker can assist with only if allowed by her agency?
    A. Hip abduction and adduction
    B. Neck exercises
    C. Knee exercises
    D. Shoulder exercises

22. When you move a joint during range-of-motion exercises and the client complains of pain, what should you do?
    A. Ask the nurse to give pain medication before you continue.
    B. Do not force the joint to the point of pain.
    C. Stop doing any range-of-motion exercises with the client.
    D. Push slightly past the point where pain occurs to restore movement.

23. When range-of-motion exercises are performed, how often should each exercise be repeated?
    A. Once
    B. Twice
    C. Five times or according to the care plan
    D. Until the client complains of being tired

24. Improperly fitted crutches can cause:
    A. Falls
    B. Back pain and nerve damage
    C. Injuries to the underarms and palms
    D. All of the above

25. Which statement about contractures is correct?
    A. Contractures are reversible with exercise.
    B. Contractures can form in as little as 48 to 72 hours.
    C. Contractures cannot form in the neck.
    D. Bed cradles prevent contractures.

Copyright © 2018 Elsevier Canada, a division of Reed Elsevier Canada, Ltd.

MATCHING

Match the following statements with the correct terms related to exercise and activity.

26. _____ Support placed to prevent external rotation of hips and legs

27. _____ Swinging bar on overbed frame that allows the client to move in bed

28. _____ Decrease in size or wasting away of tissue

29. _____ Turning downward

30. _____ Device placed to keep soles of feet flush against it with feet in flexed position

31. _____ Abnormal shortening of a muscle

32. _____ Sections of plywood used to prevent mattress from sagging

33. _____ Footdrop

34. _____ Exercise of all joints of the body

A. Footboard

B. Contracture

C. Atrophy

D. Bed board

E. Plantar flexion

F. Trochanter roll

G. Trapeze

H. Range-of-motion exercises

I. Pronation

Copyright © 2018 Elsevier Canada, a division of Reed Elsevier Canada, Ltd.

Match each movement with the correct description.

35. _____ Turn head from side to side

36. _____ Turn hand so palm is down

37. _____ Turn hand toward thumb

38. _____ Bend arm so that same-side shoulder is touched

39. _____ Pull foot forward and push down on heel at same time

40. _____ Move straight arm away from side of body

41. _____ Turn foot down or point the toes

42. _____ Move head to the right and to the left

43. _____ Touch each fingertip to thumb

44. _____ Turn hand toward little finger

45. _____ Move forearm toward head

46. _____ Move leg toward the other leg

47. _____ Straighten fingers so fingers, hand, and wrist are straight

48. _____ Bend the hand back

49. _____ Turn inside of foot up and outside down

50. _____ Turn leg inward

A. Abduction

B. Adduction

C. Flexion

D. Internal rotation

E. Extension

F. Hyperextension

G. Rotation

H. Lateral flexion

I. External rotation

J. Pronation

K. Supination

L. Opposition

M. Plantar flexion

N. Dorsiflexion

O. Radial flexion

P. Ulnar flexion

Match the following types of range-of-motion exercises with the correct definition.

51. _____ Someone moves the client's joints through ROM exercises

52. _____ The client does the exercises with the help of another person

53. _____ The client does the exercises by himself

A. Active

B. Passive

C. Active-assisted

Copyright © 2018 Elsevier Canada, a division of Reed Elsevier Canada, Ltd.

FILL IN THE BLANKS

54. Describe the following types of bed rest:
    a. Bed rest

    _____

    b. Strict bed rest

    _____

    c. Bed rest with commode privileges

    _____

    d. Bed rest with bathroom privileges

    _____

55. What problem can be prevented by using a footboard? _____

56. Depending on the child's activity limits, almost any play activity promotes _____ _____ in children.

57. What device is used to safely transfer or ambulate the person?

    _____

58. Why do you ease a client who is falling onto the floor instead of trying to stop the fall?

    _____

59. A client using a cane should follow these steps:
    a. Step A

    _____

    b. Step B

    _____

    c. Step C

    _____

Copyright © 2018 Elsevier Canada, a division of Reed Elsevier Canada, Ltd.

CROSSWORD

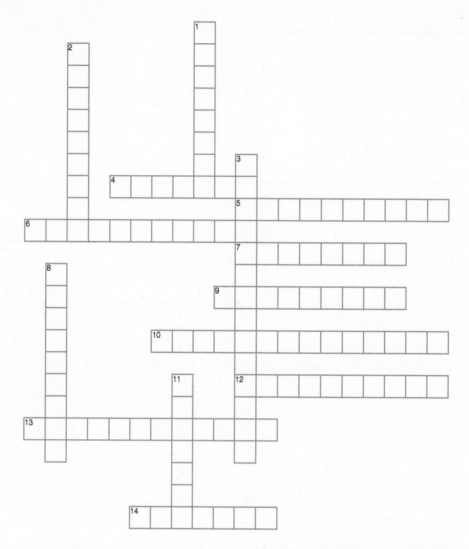

Across

4. Decrease in size or a wasting away of tissue

5. Turning downward

6. Lack of joint mobility caused by abnormal shortening of a muscle

7. Turning the joint

9. Straightening of a body part

10. Movement of a joint to the extent possible without causing pain (*3 words*)

12. Turning upward

13. Bending the toes and foot up at the ankles

14. Brief loss of consciousness; fainting

Down

1. Foot falls down at the ankle (permanent plantar flexion)

2. Moving a body part toward the midline of the body

3. Excessive straightening of a body part

8. Moving a body part away from the midline of the body

11. Bending a body part

Copyright © 2018 Elsevier Canada, a division of Reed Elsevier Canada, Ltd.

Rehabilitation Care

TRUE OR FALSE

Circle T for true, or circle F for false.

1. **T   F**   A disability does not affect the client's psychological well-being. It is only a physical problem.

2. **T   F**   Rehabilitation begins by preventing complications.

3. **T   F**   Rehabilitation often takes less time for older clients than for clients in other age groups.

4. **T   F**   Health care workers as well as the client and family members are part of the rehabilitation team.

5. **T   F**   Restorative care is usually provided by the family physician.

6. **T   F**   The goal of using a prosthesis is that it should be like the missing body part in function, appearance, or both.

7. **T   F**   Rehabilitation can occur in the community as well as in long-term care settings.

8. **T   F**   Good skin care is important in rehabilitation as it can prevent further disability and illness.

9. **T   F**   An electric toothbrush may make brushing the teeth more difficult for a client who has limited arm movement.

10. **T   F**   The home is assessed by the rehabilitation team after a client goes home.

MULTIPLE RESPONSE

From the list below, choose all of the correct answers.

11. Which of the following are goals of rehabilitation?
    A. To restore function as much as possible for each client
    B. To improve a client's functional abilities
    C. To cure diseases
    D. To teach clients new skills
    E. To prevent further disability and illness

12. Examples of orthoses include which of the following?
    A. Splints
    B. Foot support
    C. Transfer belt
    D. Knee and back braces

13. Common health problems requiring rehabilitation include which of the following?
    A. Acquired brain injury
    B. Alcoholism
    C. Amputation
    D. Brain tumour
    E. Poor nutrition
    F. Cerebral palsy
    G. Chronic obstructive pulmonary disease

14. How can you improve the quality of life for a client with a disability?
    A. Allow the client to practise skills in private.
    B. Share information about a client's progress with other clients.
    C. Allow for personal choice whenever possible.
    D. Focus on the positive.
    E. Offer praise only when goals are met.
    F. Never force clients to do more than they are able.
    G. Perform activities of daily living for the client as much as possible.

MULTIPLE CHOICE

Circle the correct answer.

15. An orthotic is:
    A. An artificial replacement for missing body parts
    B. The process of correcting a deformity
    C. An apparatus worn for support
    D. The process of restoring a client to the highest level of functioning possible

16. Rehabilitation:
    A. Is often slow and frustrating
    B. Occurs quickly
    C. Is carried out only in a hospital
    D. Does not involve the family

17. Occupational therapists on the rehabilitation team:
    A. Lead and coordinate rehabilitation
    B. Assess the performance of activities of daily living
    C. Test speech
    D. Coordinate home care

18. Social workers on the rehabilitation team:
    A. Provide counselling
    B. Help with physiotherapy
    C. Coordinate and provide care at every stage
    D. Evaluate strength

19. Which member of the rehabilitation team assesses the client's performance of activities of daily living?
    A. The physiotherapist
    B. The occupational therapist
    C. The case manager
    D. The speech–language pathologist

Copyright © 2018 Elsevier Canada, a division of Reed Elsevier Canada, Ltd.

MATCHING

Match the following words with the correct definitions.

20. _____ Process of restoring a person to the highest possible level of function

21. _____ Self-care activities performed to remain independence

22. _____ Helps a person regain health and strength

A.   Activities of daily living

B.   Independence

C.   Rehabilitation

FILL IN THE BLANKS

23. Rehabilitation can occur in different settings. List some of the settings.

   a. _____

   b. _____

   c. _____

   d. _____

Copyright © 2018 Elsevier Canada, a division of Reed Elsevier Canada, Ltd.

Nutrition and Fluids

TRUE OR FALSE

Circle T for true, or circle F for false.

1. T   F   The body becomes swollen if too much sugar is retained.

2. T   F   When a healthy client eats more sodium than the body needs, it will be excreted.

3. T   F   A client with diabetes will retain salt in the body.

4. T   F   When a client has diabetes, sugar builds up in the bloodstream.

5. T   F   When a client is placed on a diabetic diet, only three meals each day are allowed.

6. T   F   A client on a clear-liquid diet is allowed water, gelatin, and popsicles.

7. T   F   A client who has constipation may be helped by a high-fibre diet.

8. T   F   Many special diets involve between-meal nourishments such as crackers and milk.

9. T   F   There are four calories in 1 g of carbohydrate.

10. T   F   One gram of fat contains nine calories.

11. T   F   One gram of protein contains five calories.

12. T   F   Chopped foods may be added to an infant's diet at about 5 months of age.

13. T   F   Clients from India generally do not eat beef..

14. T   F   Clients who must eat in bed should be positioned in the supine position.

15. T   F   A decrease in saliva may cause difficulty swallowing.

16. T   F   Decreased peristalsis results in slower emptying of the stomach and colon, causing flatulence and constipation.

17. T   F   Cooked fruits and vegetables may be eaten to prevent constipation.

18. **T**   **F**   Too much sodium in the diet causes the body to retain more water.

19. **T**   **F**   When a client is on a sodium-restricted diet, the only food group without restrictions is fruits and vegetables.

20. **T**   **F**   Clients with diabetes must eat at regular times to maintain their cholesterol levels.

21. **T**   **F**   When a client has dysphagia, the care plan might indicate that he is on a puréed diet.

22. **T**   **F**   The daily minimum amount of water required for an adult to survive is 800 mL.

23. **T**   **F**   To maintain normal fluid balance, a client needs 2000–2500 mL of fluids each day.

24. **T**   **F**   An older client should increase calorie intake, as more calories are needed as we age.

25. **T**   **F**   An older client should increase fluid intake to aid in digestion, kidney function, chewing, and swallowing.

26. **T**   **F**   An older client should increase protein intake for tissue growth and repair.

27. **T**   **F**   An older client should decrease soft bulk to prevent constipation.

28. **T**   **F**   An older client should decrease intake of fried, fatty foods as these are hard to digest.

MULTIPLE RESPONSE

From the list below, choose all of the correct answers.

29. Which of the following dietary guidelines are recommended for healthy eating?
    A. Select dietary choices only from one food group.
    B. Emphasize cereals, breads, other grain products, vegetables, and fruit.
    C. Choose higher-fat dairy products, leaner meats, and foods prepared with little or no fat.
    D. Participate in regular physical activity and healthy eating.
    E. Limit salt, alcohol, and caffeine.

30. In what ways, other than positioning, can you help clients to get ready for meals?
    A. Assist with elimination and hand hygiene.
    B. Change clothing and provide clean linens if necessary.
    C. Be sure dentures, eyeglasses, and hearing aids are in place.
    D. Decide their menu choices.
    E. Make the setting attractive.

31. Which of the following actions are important for safety and comfort when feeding a client?
    A. Provide a relaxed mood.
    B. Provide time and privacy to pray.
    C. Use a fork to feed the client.
    D. Offer larger portions.
    E. Offer fluids during the meal.
    F. Engage the client in conversation.
    G. Stand while you are feeding the client.
    H. Encourage the client to feed herself.

Copyright © 2018 Elsevier Canada, a division of Reed Elsevier Canada, Ltd.

32. Which of the following are common causes of dehydration?
    A. Adequate fluid intake
    B. Vomiting
    C. Diarrhea
    D. Bleeding
    E. Excess sweating
    F. Decreased urine production

33. Which of the following food groups are included in *Eating Well with Canada's Food Guide*?
    A. Grain products
    B. Vegetables and fruit
    C. Sugar and other sweets
    D. Milk products
    E. Meat and alternatives

MULTIPLE CHOICE

Circle the correct answer.

34. Why are carbohydrates important in the diet?
    A. They supply products for tissue growth and repair.
    B. They provide energy and bulk for bowel elimination.
    C. They provide energy and flavour.
    D. They supply vitamins that are needed daily.

35. What can you give a client who has an order for NPO?
    A. Unlimited fluids
    B. No food or fluids
    C. Small amounts of fluids
    D. Only clear liquids

36. What effect may cultural and religious beliefs have on nutrition?
    A. Certain types of food may be restricted.
    B. Methods of preparation may be part of beliefs.
    C. Certain foods are eaten, and others are avoided.
    D. All of the above may be part of beliefs.

37. Which of these foods would be included as liquid intake?
    A. Spaghetti sauce
    B. Yogourt
    C. Cottage cheese
    D. Beef stew

38. Which of the following statements describes assistive dining?
    A. One client is fed by one support worker to reduce stimulation.
    B. Food is placed on platters or dishes, and the clients serve themselves.
    C. Clients are served food at the table as in a restaurant.
    D. Four clients are seated at a horseshoe-shaped table and are fed by one support worker.

Use the following conversion table to answer questions 39 to 46.
1 oz = 30 mL (cc)
1 cup = 250 mL (cc)
1 quart = 1 000 mL (cc) or 1 litre
1 cc = 1 mL

39. A 6-oz cup of coffee = how many mLs?
    A. 160 mL
    B. 180 mL
    C. 170 mL
    D. 200 mL

40. 8 oz of milk = how many mLs?
    A. 200 mL
    B. 260 mL
    C. 240 mL
    D. 230 mL

41. 1 quart of water = how many mLs?
    A. 1 000 mL
    B. 900 mL
    C. 1 020 mL
    D. 1 010 mL

42. 2 cups of tea = how many mLs?
    A. 460 mL
    B. 440 mL
    C. 480 mL
    D. 400 mL

Copyright © 2018 Elsevier Canada, a division of Reed Elsevier Canada, Ltd.

43. 4 oz of gelatin = how many mLs?
    A.   100 mL
    B.   120 mL
    C.   130 mL
    D.   140 mL

44. 5 oz of orange juice = how many mLs?
    A.   150 mL
    B.   130 mL
    C.   170 mL
    D.   140 mL

45. 12 oz of broth = how many mLs?
    A.   340 mL
    B.   380 mL
    C.   360 mL
    D.   320 mL

46. A half-cup of sherbet = how many mLs?
    A.   100 mL
    B.   110 mL
    C.   120 mL
    D.   130 mL

MATCHING

Match the nutrient with the reason it is important to good health.

47. _____ Needed for tooth and bone formation

48. _____ Needed for tissue growth and repair

49. _____ Provides energy and adds flavour

50. _____ Provides energy and fibre for elimination

51. _____ Does not provide calories but is needed for certain body functions

A.   Protein

B.   Carbohydrates

C.   Fats

D.   Vitamins

E.   Minerals

Copyright © 2018 Elsevier Canada, a division of Reed Elsevier Canada, Ltd.

Match the correct vitamin with its major function.

52. _____ Healthy eyes, healthy skin and mucous
membranes, protein and carbohydrate metabolism

53. _____ Formation of substances that hold tissues
together

54. _____ Formation of red blood cells, nervous system
functioning

55. _____ Blood clotting

56. _____ Normal reproduction

57. _____ Growth, vision, healthy hair and skin

58. _____ Muscle tone, nerve function, digestion

59. _____ Protein, fat, and carbohydrate metabolism

60. _____ Formation of red blood cells, functioning of
intestine

61. _____ Absorption and metabolism of calcium and
phosphorus, healthy bones

A. Vitamin A

B. Thiamine

C. Riboflavin

D. Niacin

E. Vitamin B_{12}

F. Folic acid

G. Ascorbic acid

H. Vitamin D

I. Vitamin E

J. Vitamin K

Match the correct mineral with its major function.

62. _____ Formation of bone and teeth; use of protein,
fats, and carbohydrates

63. _____ Thyroid gland function, growth, metabolism

64. _____ Fluid balance, nerve function, muscle function

65. _____ Formation of bone and teeth, blood clotting,
muscle contraction

66. _____ Enabling red blood cells to carry oxygen

67. _____ Nerve function, muscle contraction, heart
function

A. Calcium

B. Phosphorus

C. Iron

D. Iodine

E. Sodium

F. Potassium

Copyright © 2018 Elsevier Canada, a division of Reed Elsevier Canada, Ltd.

Match each of the following situations with the appropriate special diet.

68. _____ First diet most clients can tolerate after surgery

69. _____ Constipation and colon disorders

70. _____ Weight gain and certain thyroid imbalances

71. _____ Heart disease, gallbladder disease

72. _____ Burns, high fever, infection

A.   High-protein

B.   Fat-controlled/low-cholesterol

C.   Clear-liquid

D.   High-calorie

E.   High-fibre

Match each of the following food items to the correct food group.

73. _____ Crackers

74. _____ Kidney beans

75. _____ Potatoes

76. _____ Ice milk

77. _____ Chocolate bar

A.   Vegetables and fruit

B.   Grain products

C.   Meat and alternatives

D.   Milk products

E.   Other foods

Match each of the following food items to the correct food group.

78. _____ Pineapple chunks

79. _____ Peanut butter

80. _____ Oatmeal

81. _____ Butter tart

82. _____ Sour cream

A.   Vegetables and fruit

B.   Grain products

C.   Meat and alternatives

D.   Milk products

E.   Other foods

FILL IN THE BLANKS

83. How many servings of meat, poultry, or fish are recommended daily for an older adult? _____
    _____

84. If an older client must avoid high-fibre foods, what foods may be eaten to prevent constipation?
    _____

Copyright © 2018 Elsevier Canada, a division of Reed Elsevier Canada, Ltd.

85. Why are the following actions important for safety and comfort when feeding a client?
    a. Provide a relaxed mood

    _____

    b. Provide time and privacy to pray

    _____

    c. Use spoon to feed

    _____

    d. Offer small portions (spoon that is 1/3 tsp full)

    _____

    e. Offer fluids during meal

    _____

    f. Engage in conversation

    _____

    g. Sit so you face client

    _____

    h. Encourage the client to feed himself or herself

    _____

86. Should an older client increase or decrease these dietary elements? Why?
    a. Calories _____

       Why? _____

    b. Fluids _____

       Why? _____

    c. Protein _____

       Why? _____

    d. Soft bulk _____

       Why? _____

    e. Fried, fatty foods _____

       Why? _____

Copyright © 2018 Elsevier Canada, a division of Reed Elsevier Canada, Ltd.

LABELLING

87. Label the plate with numbers so that you could describe the location of food to a client who is blind.

    a. Where would you tell the client to find the meat? _____

    b. Where would you tell the client to find the baked potato? _____

Copyright © 2018 Elsevier Canada, a division of Reed Elsevier Canada, Ltd.

Enteral Nutrition and Intravenous Therapy

TRUE OR FALSE

Circle T for true, or circle F for false.

1. **T** **F**   During a scheduled tube feeding, 400 mL (13.5 fluid oz) is usually given over 20 minutes.

2. **T** **F**   Formula for feeding tubes should be heated.

3. **T** **F**   The risk of regurgitation is less with nasointestinal tubes than with other types of tubes.

4. **T** **F**   Mouth care is not important when clients are NPO.

5. **T** **F**   An intravenous (IV) site on the back of the hand is in a central venous site.

6. **T** **F**   Support workers should check the placement of the feeding tube before each feeding.

7. **T** **F**   You should clean the client's nose and nostrils around the feeding tube every 4 to 8 hours.

8. **T** **F**   Support workers are responsible for maintaining IV therapy.

9. **T** **F**   Notify your supervisor immediately if there is any leaking of fluid from the IV site.

10. **T** **F**   Clients should be sitting or in the semi-Fowler's position during tube feedings.

11. **T** **F**   Scheduled enteral feedings are usually given four times a day.

12. **T** **F**   Continuous enteral feedings require an electric feeding pump.

13. **T** **F**   When a client is receiving an enteral feeding, he or she is in a supine position for at least 1–2 hours.

Copyright © 2018 Elsevier Canada, a division of Reed Elsevier Canada, Ltd.

14.   T   F   Frequent oral care can help a client with a feeding tube feel more comfortable.

15.   T   F   The left-side-lying position should be avoided when a client is receiving enteral nutrition as this position prevents the stomach from emptying.

MULTIPLE RESPONSE

From the list below, choose all of the correct answers.

16.   What conditions may require a client to have a feeding tube?
   A.   Cancers of the head, neck, and esophagus
   B.   Coma
   C.   Dysphagia caused by paralysis
   D.   Trauma or surgery to the face, head, mouth, or neck
   E.   Dementia

17.   What can cause the feeding tube to move?
   A.   Coughing
   B.   Sneezing
   C.   Vomiting
   D.   Talking
   E.   Suctioning
   F.   Poor positioning

18.   When you care for a client with a feeding tube at home, which of the following is the support worker allowed to do?
   A.   Insert feeding tubes
   B.   Test the position of the tube
   C.   Give the first dose of a tube feeding
   D.   Pour formula into a feeding bag
   E.   Start feed after placement of tube has been verified by the nurse

19.   What should be reported to the nurse if the client is receiving a tube feeding?
   A.   Nausea or vomiting
   B.   Discomfort during the tube feeding
   C.   Diarrhea
   D.   Distended abdomen
   E.   Coughing
   F.   Complaints of indigestion or heartburn
   G.   Redness, swelling, drainage, odour, or pain at the ostomy site
   H.   Normal temperature
   I.   Signs and symptoms of respiratory distress
   J.   Complaints of flatulence

20.   A client may receive IV therapy to:
   A.   Receive fluids
   B.   Receive minerals and vitamins
   C.   Receive sugar for energy
   D.   Receive blood
   E.   Receive oral medications
   F.   Receive hyperalimentation (a solution highly concentrated with nutrients)

21.   What safety measures must be followed when the client has an IV?
   A.   Follow Standard Practices.
   B.   Move the needle or catheter if the IV is not running.
   C.   Follow the safety measures for restraints if the nurse restrains the extremity to prevent the needle or catheter from moving.
   D.   Protect the IV bag, tubing, and needle or catheter when ambulating the client.
   E.   Assist the client with turning and repositioning.
   F.   Move the bag to the side of the bed on which the client is lying, allowing enough slack in the tubing.
   G.   Notify your supervisor immediately if bleeding occurs from the insertion site.
   H.   Notify your supervisor immediately if you notice signs or symptoms of complications.

Copyright © 2018 Elsevier Canada, a division of Reed Elsevier Canada, Ltd.

22. What signs and symptoms indicate that there is a problem with an IV site?
    A.   Bleeding
    B.   Puffiness or swelling
    C.   Pale or reddened skin
    D.   Complaints of pain at or above the IV site
    E.   Hot or cold skin near the site

23. What signs and symptoms indicate that there is a systemic problem with an IV?
    A.   Fever
    B.   Itching
    C.   Drop in blood pressure
    D.   Bradycardia
    E.   Regular pulse
    F.   Pink skin
    G.   Changes in mental function
    H.   Loss of consciousness
    I.   Difficulty breathing
    J.   Increasing urine output
    K.   Chest pain
    L.   Nausea

MULTIPLE CHOICE

Circle the correct answer.

24. Which of the following describes a gastrostomy tube?
    A.   A tube is inserted through a surgical opening into the stomach.
    B.   A tube is inserted through the nose and into the stomach.
    C.   An opening is made into the middle part of the small intestine.
    D.   A tube is inserted through the nose and into the duodenum.

25. What responsibility does the support worker have if a client is being fed through a tube?
    A.   Removing the tube after each feeding
    B.   Giving clear liquids by mouth
    C.   Assisting the nurse in giving feedings
    D.   Avoiding giving mouth care

26. Clients who cannot chew or swallow often receive nutrition by:
    A.   Enteral nutrition
    B.   IV feedings
    C.   A liquid diet
    D.   A puréed diet

27. Support workers are responsible for:
    A.   Inserting feeding tubes
    B.   Testing the position of the tube
    C.   Giving the first dose of a tube feeding
    D.   Providing personal care to the client

28. Physicians order IV therapy to:
    A.   Replace minerals and vitamins lost due to illness
    B.   Administer medications
    C.   Administer blood
    D.   Do all of the above

29. A sign of an IV therapy complication is:
    A.   Vomiting
    B.   Swelling around the site
    C.   Indigestion
    D.   Diarrhea

Copyright © 2018 Elsevier Canada, a division of Reed Elsevier Canada, Ltd.

MATCHING

Match the type of feeding tube with the correct gastrointestinal tract route.

30. _____ Gastrostomy tube

31. _____ Percutaneous endoscopic gastrostomy [PEG] tube

32. _____ Jejunostomy tube

33. _____ Nasointestinal tube

34. _____ Nasogastric tube

A. Through the nose into the stomach

B. Through the nose into the small intestine

C. Into the stomach through a surgically created opening

D. Into the intestines through a surgically created opening

E. Into the stomach through a surgically created opening; an endoscope is fed through the mouth and into the stomach

You may care for clients who have IVs in different sites. Match the site where each of these IVs would be inserted.

35. _____ Peripheral

36. _____ Scalp

37. _____ Central venous sites

38. _____ Peripherally inserted central catheter (PICC)

A. In the subclavian vein or the internal jugular vein

B. In the cephalic or basilic veins in the arm

C. On the back of the hand, in the forearm, or in the crease of the elbow

D. On the head

FILL IN THE BLANKS

39. How do these measures help clients with feeding tubes feel more comfortable?
    a. Hard candy or gum

    _____

    b. Lubricant for lips

    _____

    c. Cleaning of nose and nostrils every 4 to 8 hours

    _____

    d. Frequent oral hygiene

    _____

Personal Hygiene

TRUE OR FALSE

Circle T for true, or circle F for false.

1. T F Soap dries the skin, especially in older clients.

2. T F The support worker decides what skin care products to use when giving a client a bath.

3. T F Plain water may be used for the bath when the skin is very dry.

4. T F Bath oils and lotions are used to clean the skin.

5. T F Adjust the water temperature and pressure before the client gets in the shower.

6. T F Illness and disease can cause a bad taste in the mouth.

7. T F Some medications and diseases can cause a white coating on the tongue.

8. T F Children should learn to brush their teeth at about age 5.

9. T F Cold water should not be used to clean or store dentures because it may cause them to warp.

10. T F When you are giving mouth care to an unconscious client, it is important to position the client on his or her back to avoid aspiration.

11. T F If an older client with dementia resists your effort to assist with hygiene, you may find ways to work with the client in the care plan.

12. T F Older clients with dementia sometimes become agitated and combative during bathing procedures as they do not understand what is happening or why.

13. T F The tub or shower should be cleaned before using to prevent the spread of microbes and infection.

14. T F The cleanest part of the perineal area is the anal region.

MULTIPLE RESPONSE

From the list below, choose all of the correct answers.

15. When should oral hygiene be performed?
    A. Upon awakening
    B. After each meal
    C. Every other day
    D. At bedtime
    E. Before meals (if the client wishes)

16. When giving oral care, what observations should you report to the nurse?
    A. Dry, cracked, swollen, or blistered lips
    B. Redness, swelling, irritation, sores, or white patches in the mouth or on the tongue
    C. Bleeding, swelling, or redness of the gums
    D. Loose teeth
    E. Rough, sharp, or chipped areas on dentures
    F. Complaints of pain or discomfort

17. What are reasons for bathing a client?
    A. To clean the skin and mucous membranes of the genital and anal areas
    B. To remove microbes, dead skin, perspiration, and excess oils
    C. To refresh and relax the client
    D. To stimulate circulation and exercise body parts

18. How can the support worker help the client with dementia to tolerate a bath?
    A. Not rushing the client
    B. Using a loud, firm voice
    C. Diverting the client's attention
    D. Calming the client and, if the client resists, trying again later

19. When giving a tub bath or shower, what safety measures will help to prevent falls?
    A. Dry the bathroom or shower room floor.
    B. Check handrails, grab bars, hydraulic lifts, and other safety aids to ensure they are in working order.
    C. Place a bath mat inside tubs or showers without a nonskid surface.
    D. Place needed items out of the client's reach.
    E. Place the call bell within the client's reach.
    F. Have the client use towel bars when getting in and out of the tub or shower.
    G. Do not use bath oils because they make surfaces slippery.
    H. Keep bar soap in the dish to prevent the client from slipping on it.
    I. Do not leave weak or unsteady clients unattended.
    J. Stay within hearing distance if the client can be left alone.

20. What observations should you make and report when you give a client a bath?
    A. The colour of the skin, lips, nail beds, and sclera
    B. The location and description of rashes
    C. Normal skin
    D. Bruises or open skin areas
    E. Pale or reddened areas, particularly over bony parts
    F. Drainage or bleeding from wounds or body openings
    G. Swelling of the feet and legs
    H. Corns or calluses on the feet
    I. Skin temperature
    J. Complaints of pain or discomfort

Copyright © 2018 Elsevier Canada, a division of Reed Elsevier Canada, Ltd.

21. What areas are bathed when giving a partial bath?
    A. Face
    B. Hands
    C. Underarms
    D. Feet
    E. Back
    F. Buttocks
    G. Perineal area

22. What are reasons a complete bed bath may be ordered?
    A. The client is conscious.
    B. The client is paralyzed.
    C. The client is in a cast or traction.
    D. The client is weak from illness or surgery.

23. Back massages should not be given to clients with:
    A. Certain heart diseases
    B. Back injuries
    C. Back surgeries
    D. Skin diseases
    E. Some lung disorders

MULTIPLE CHOICE

Circle the correct answer.

24. When giving oral care, why should you wear gloves?
    A. You will have contact with the mucous membranes.
    B. The gums may bleed.
    C. There may be harmful bacteria (pathogens) in the mouth.
    D. All of the above are correct.

25. How often should mouth care be given to an unconscious client?
    A. Once a day
    B. Once each shift
    C. After every meal
    D. Every 2 hours

26. Why should you avoid using bath oils when giving a tub bath or shower?
    A. They make the tub or floor slippery.
    B. They may be irritating to the skin.
    C. They will cause dryness of the skin.
    D. They may collect in skin folds and cause skin breakdown.

27. Before being given a bath, the client should be assisted to the bathroom or offered the commode, bedpan, or urinal because:
    A. This will prevent incontinence during the bath
    B. Bathing stimulates urination
    C. It will prevent skin breakdown during the bath
    D. It will prevent soiling after the bath

28. About how long should a back massage last?
    A. 1 to 2 minutes
    B. 3 to 5 minutes
    C. 6 to 8 minutes
    D. At least 10 minutes

29. What is one reason to provide perineal care at least once a day?
    A. To prevent the growth of microbes that can cause infection
    B. To prevent incontinence
    C. To prevent pain
    D. To provide exercise

30. Which of the following is the correct way to wash the perineal area?
    A. Wash from the anal area toward the urethra.
    B. Wash in a circular motion from the outside to the inside.
    C. Wash from the urethra to the anal area.
    D. Wash back and forth over the entire area several times.

Copyright © 2018 Elsevier Canada, a division of Reed Elsevier Canada, Ltd.

31. When should the bathwater be changed during a complete bed bath?
    A. After washing the chest and abdomen if the water is soapy or cool
    B. Before washing the feet and legs
    C. After giving perineal care
    D. Only if it is soapy or cool

32. Which of these steps is not correct when giving perineal care to a male client?
    A. Retract the foreskin of the uncircumcised male.
    B. Wash the tip of the penis starting at the urethral opening and working outward.
    C. Clean the shaft of the penis with firm, downward strokes.
    D. Leave the foreskin retracted at the end of the procedure.

FILL IN THE BLANKS

33. What causes these problems in the oral cavity?
    a. Bad taste

    _____

    b. White coating on tongue

    _____

    c. Redness and swelling of tongue and mouth

    _____

    d. Dry mouth

    _____

34. When you are cleaning dentures, why do you fill the sink or basin with water and line it with a towel? _____

35. Hot water should not be used to clean or store dentures because it may cause them to

    _____.

36. What are the reasons the teeth should be flossed?

    a. _____

    b. _____

37. Dentures are stored in _____

38. When giving mouth care to an unconscious client, it is important to turn the person

    _____ to

    prevent _____ .

39. Why are the following rules important when bathing a client?
    a. Keep soap in dish between lathering

    _____

    b. Rinse the skin

    _____

    c. Pat the skin dry

    _____

    d. Bathe the skin whenever urine and feces are present

    _____

40. How can you provide for warmth during a bath?

    a. _____

    b. _____

41. Lower water temperature for bathing is

    important for _____ because they

    have _____ .

42. Why is the water temperature for a bed bath 43.3° to 46.1°C?

    _____

43. When washing and drying the chest during a bed bath, what steps are taken to avoid exposing the client?

    a. _____

    b. _____

    c. _____

Copyright © 2018 Elsevier Canada, a division of Reed Elsevier Canada, Ltd.

44. The cleanest area in the perineal area is the
_____ and
the dirtiest area is the _____
_____ .

45. When giving perineal care, what observations should be reported to the nurse?

a. _____

b. _____

c. _____

LABELLING

46. Using arrows, show the directions in which the teeth should be brushed.

47. Using an arrow, show the direction used to clean the eyes while giving a bed bath.

48. Draw lines with arrows to show the direction your hands move when giving a backrub.

Copyright © 2018 Elsevier Canada, a division of Reed Elsevier Canada, Ltd.

Grooming and Dressing

TRUE OR FALSE

Circle T for true, or circle F for false.

1. T F How the hair looks has no effect on the client's well-being.

2. T F When brushing hair, start at the scalp and brush to the hair ends.

3. T F If hair is tangled and matted, first start to brush at the scalp and brush to the ends.

4. T F When caring for adolescents, style hair in a manner that pleases the client and parents.

5. T F Older clients need to shampoo more frequently because of decreased oil gland secretion.

6. T F A female client may want you to shave coarse facial hair.

7. T F When you are shaving the face, the client's skin should be loose.

8. T F Fingernails should be trimmed with scissors.

9. T F Brushing and combing are important to prevent tangles in long hair.

10. T F Garbage bags can be used to make a plastic trough to wash the hair of a client in bed at home.

11. T F When you are giving foot care, you should treat corns and blisters.

12. T F Poor circulation to feet and toes can be caused by diabetes or vascular disease.

13. T F Gangrene and amputation are serious complications of foot injuries.

14. T F The best time to clean and trim fingernails is right after they have been soaked or a client has been bathed.

15. T F Shampooing at the sink or on a stretcher is difficult for people with limited range of motion in their legs and hips.

Copyright © 2018 Elsevier Canada, a division of Reed Elsevier Canada, Ltd.

16. **T   F**   Standard Practices should always be followed when shaving a client to prevent contact with their blood from a nick or cut.

17. **T   F**   An adolescent may need frequent shampooing because oil gland secretion decreases during puberty, resulting in hair that is drier than normal.

18. **T   F**   You can soften the skin before shaving by applying a warm towel to the face for a few minutes.

MULTIPLE RESPONSE

From the list below, choose all of the correct answers.

19. What specific measures are needed to comb curly, coarse, or dry hair?
   A. Use a wide-tooth comb.
   B. Wet the hair or use cooking oil to make combing easier.
   C. Begin at the neckline and comb upward, lifting and fluffing hair outward.

20. How can client safety and comfort be achieved with different methods of shampooing?
   A. During a shower or bath, support the back of the client's head with a pillow while shampooing the client's hair.
   B. If the client must lean forward, have him place a folded washcloth over his eyes, and support his forehead with one hand as you shampoo with the other hand.
   C. If the client is in a wheelchair, have her lean back over the sink. Place a folded towel over the sink edge to protect her neck.
   D. If the client is in a wheelchair, make sure it is securely locked in place.
   E. If the client is on a stretcher, his hair should not be shampooed.
   F. If the client is in bed, place a shampoo tray under her head to protect the linens and mattress.

21. If nicks or cuts occur when shaving a client, you should:
   A. Apply direct pressure to the nick or cut
   B. Apply pressure around the nick or cut but never apply pressure directly to the cut itself
   C. Report the nick or cut to your supervisor at once

22. Observations that should be reported to the nurse during foot care include:
   A. Soft, pink, intact skin
   B. Very dry skin
   C. Foot odours
   D. Cracks or breaks in the skin, especially between the toes
   E. Ingrown nails
   F. Loose nails
   G. Reddened, irritated, or calloused areas on the feet, heels, or ankles
   H. No drainage or bleeding
   I. Change in colour or texture of nails, especially black, thick, or brittle nails
   J. Corns, bunions, or blisters

23. When the client requests a shampoo, you should:
   A. Shampoo the client's hair while she is in bed to avoid tiring her out
   B. Follow the client's care plan
   C. Explain that shampooing is not your job
   D. Wear gloves if the client has scalp lesions or head lice

MULTIPLE CHOICE

Circle the correct answer.

24. Microbes (or bacteria) can be found on dirty:
   A. Shoes
   B. Socks
   C. Feet
   D. All of the above

Copyright © 2018 Elsevier Canada, a division of Reed Elsevier Canada, Ltd.

25. A client has long hair. Which procedure cannot be done?
    A. Daily brushing and combing
    B. Shampooing
    C. Cutting the hair to remove tangles and matting
    D. Braiding or styling

26. A female client in a long-term care facility has her hair done weekly at the beauty shop. During her shower, you should:
    A. Wash her hair as usual
    B. Protect her hair with a shower cap
    C. Be careful not to get water on her hair
    D. Wrap a towel around her head to protect her hair

27. Which of these should you wear when you are shaving a client?
    A. Gown
    B. Gloves
    C. Mask
    D. Gown, gloves, and mask

28. Which of these statements is correct about dressing or undressing a client?
    A. Remove clothing from the affected side first.
    B. Put clothing on the affected side first.
    C. Put clothing on the unaffected side first.
    D. Remove clothing from the side farthest away from you first.

29. Which of these steps is correct when you change the gown of a client receiving intravenous (IV) therapy?
    A. Remove the gown from the arm with the IV first.
    B. Gather up the sleeve of the arm with the IV and slide it over the IV site and tubing.
    C. Turn off the IV and disconnect it temporarily while changing the gown.
    D. Put the gown on the arm without the IV first.

MATCHING

Match each of the following descriptions to the correct term related to personal care.

30. _____ Excessive body hair

31. _____ Infestation with lice in the pubic area

32. _____ Hair loss

33. _____ An infestation with lice

34. _____ You may groom hair in this manner with the person's permission

35. _____ Excessive amounts of dry, white flakes from the scalp

36. _____ Parasites that can live on different parts of the body

37. _____ You must never do this to matted or tangled hair

38. _____ Infestation of the scalp with lice

39. _____ Infestation of the body with lice

A. Cutting

B. Pediculosis pubis

C. Hirsutism

D. Pediculosis capitis

E. Dandruff

F. Pediculosis

G. Alopecia

H. Pediculosis corporis

I. Lice

J. Braiding

Copyright © 2018 Elsevier Canada, a division of Reed Elsevier Canada, Ltd.

Match each of the following descriptions to the correct term related to undressing or dressing the client.

40. When undressing a client, start with removing a pullover garment from the _____ side.

41. Prevent _____ by covering the client with a sheet.

42. You should always refrain from calling the affected side the _____ side.

43. Acronym for undressing the client is _____.

44. The _____ position is the easiest for removing clothing in bed.

45. An acronym that refers to anti-embolic stockings is _____.

A. Exposure
B. Bad
C. Affected
D. RUF
E. TED
F. Supine

FILL IN THE BLANKS

46. What should you do if the person asks to have his or her hair washed?

   _____

47. When making a plastic trough to wash hair in the bed at home, you should not use

   _____.

48. How do the following factors help to cause foot injury, infection, or odours?
   a. Dirty feet, socks, stockings

   _____

   b. Shoes and socks

   _____

   c. Poorly fitted shoes

   _____

   d. Poor circulation

   _____

   e. Diabetes, vascular diseases

   _____

   f. Trimming or cutting toenails

   _____

Copyright © 2018 Elsevier Canada, a division of Reed Elsevier Canada, Ltd.

Urinary Elimination

TRUE OR FALSE

Circle T for true, or circle F for false.

1. **T F** When assisting with normal elimination, you should practise surgical asepsis and Standard Practices.

2. **T F** Normal elimination is easier if a man can stand or a woman can sit or squat.

3. **T F** If a client has osteoporosis, pain in the joints from arthritis, or a hip replacement, a regular bedpan will be the most comfortable.

4. **T F** Incontinence is a common reason for seeking long-term care for a family member.

5. **T F** When collecting a specimen to check for a urine infection, you can use any nonsterile container.

6. **T F** A specimen container must be labelled with the client's initials, room, date, and time.

7. **T F** When you collect a urine specimen, you should tell the client not to have a bowel movement or place toilet tissue in the container.

8. **T F** The specimen container and requisition slip are taken to the laboratory in a plastic cup.

9. **T F** An adult normally produces 2 500 mL of urine every day.

10. **T F** A urinal has a hooked handle so it can be passed easily to the client.

11. **T F** When you leave a client alone to void, you should place the call bell and toilet tissue within reach.

12. **T F** After a client has voided, you should provide perineal care as needed and have the client wash his or her hands.

13. **T F** You wear gloves when emptying a bedpan or urinal to avoid contact with urine or stool.

14. **T F** If a urinary drainage bag is lower than the bladder, urine can flow back into the client's bladder and an infection can develop.

Copyright © 2018 Elsevier Canada, a division of Reed Elsevier Canada, Ltd.

15. **T   F**   Adhesive tape should never be used to secure a condom catheter because this type of tape does not stretch and may cause restricted blood flow to the penis.

16. **T   F**   Another name for urinary stones is *calculi.*

17. **T   F**   The goal of bladder training is voluntary control of urination.

18. **T   F**   When collecting a midstream urine specimen, you pass the specimen container into the urine stream (or flow) at any point during urination.

19. **T   F**   To prevent the growth of microorganisms, place a 24-hour urine specimen on ice or in a refrigerator.

20. **T   F**   Urine is strained to see if it contains crystals.

MULTIPLE RESPONSE

From the list below, choose all of the correct answers.

21. Who may use a fracture (bed) pan?
    A. Clients in casts
    B. Clients who do not like to walk to the toilet
    C. Clients with casts on their ankles
    D. Clients with limited back movement
    E. Clients with fragile bones or painful joints
    F. Clients who have recently fractured a hip

22. If a client is embarrassed about voiding with others close by, what can be done to mask the sounds?
    A. Run some water in a nearby tap
    B. Move the client to another floor or ward
    C. Flush the toilet
    D. Play music nearby

23. How can you promote relaxation and not rush a client who is voiding?
    A. Have the client practise meditation while voiding
    B. Talk to the client to provide some diversion
    C. Offer the person something to read
    D. Allow the person enough time to void

24. What measures can you take to help clients with urinary incontinence?
    A. Answer all calls for assistance promptly
    B. Encourage urination at scheduled intervals
    C. Follow the client's bladder training program
    D. Encourage the client to wear clothing with zippers and laces
    E. Encourage the client to do pelvic muscle exercises, as directed by the care plan
    F. Decrease fluid intake before bedtime
    G. Provide good skin care once a day
    H. Provide dry garments and linens
    I. Observe for signs of skin breakdown.
    J. Use incontinence products as directed by the care plan.

25. Urinary tract infections can sometimes be prevented by:
    A. Providing adequate food for the client to eat
    B. Encouraging the client to add bath oil to the tub bath
    C. Instructing the client to wear cotton undergarments
    D. Providing perineal care as needed

26. What disorders and other conditions may cause urinary incontinence?
    A. Urinary tract infections
    B. Menopause
    C. Nervous system disorders
    D. Bladder cancer
    E. Diabetes
    F. Hearing loss

Copyright © 2018 Elsevier Canada, a division of Reed Elsevier Canada, Ltd.

27. Causes of urinary incontinence include:
    A. A weakened pelvic floor
    B. An enlarged prostate
    C. Some medications
    D. Immobility
    E. The use of restraints
    F. Unanswered calls for help
    G. Confusion
    H. Certain surgeries

28. What complications can occur when a client has incontinence?
    A. Skin irritation
    B. Confusion
    C. Skin breakdown
    D. Infection

MULTIPLE CHOICE

Circle the correct answer.

29. Why is voiding in a bedside commode easier than voiding in a bedpan?
    A. It allows for a more normal position for elimination.
    B. It provides more privacy.
    C. It is more comfortable.
    D. It allows the bladder to empty completely.

30. Which of the following correctly describes catheter care?
    A. Wash the perineal area and avoid touching the catheter.
    B. Clean the meatus and the catheter with an alcohol swab.
    C. Clean the catheter from the meatus and down the catheter about 10 cm (4 in.) with soap and water.
    D. Clean the catheter with soap and water, starting about 10 cm (4 in.) below the meatus and washing toward the perineal area.

31. The urinary drainage bag should be:
    A. Secured to a bed rail
    B. Positioned below the level of the bladder at all times
    C. Placed carefully to drain on the floor
    D. Disinfected daily using bleach

32. When a client is having a 24-hour urine specimen collected, what should you do with the first voiding?
    A. Discard it.
    B. Send it to the laboratory.
    C. Place it in the large container used for saving the urine.
    D. Test it for sugar and ketones.

33. Which of these actions would be most helpful in getting a client to void?
    A. Offering to hold the urinal for the client while he is voiding.
    B. Running water in the sink while the client is sitting on the toilet.
    C. Standing next to the bed and talking quietly to the client who is urinating.
    D. Providing a glass of cold water to drink while the client is trying to void.

34. When emptying a urinary drainage bag, you maintain medical asepsis by:
    A. Using sterile gloves
    B. Placing the measuring container on a paper towel
    C. Placing the measuring container on the overbed table and stooping to read it accurately
    D. Doing all of the above

35. When straining urine, what should you do if you see particles in the strainer?
    A. Place the strainer in the container and send it to the laboratory
    B. Show it to the nurse and then discard it
    C. Send the urine and strainer to the laboratory
    D. Keep the strainer in the client's room until the doctor arrives

Copyright © 2018 Elsevier Canada, a division of Reed Elsevier Canada, Ltd.

36. When using a reagent strip to test urine, the support worker should:
   A. Send the specimen and reagent strip to the laboratory
   B. Ask the nurse to read the strip
   C. Follow the manufacturer's instructions on the container
   D. Teach the client to read the strips

MATCHING

Match each group of words with the effect that it has on urine.

37. _____ Coffee, tea, alcohol

38. _____ Diet high in salt

39. _____ Beets, blackberries

40. _____ Carrots, sweet potatoes

41. _____ Asparagus

A. Cause(s) bright yellow urine

B. Cause(s) a change in urine odour

C. Increase(s) urine production

D. Cause(s) red-coloured urine

E. Decrease(s) urine production

Match each word with its meaning.

42. _____ Painful or difficult urination

43. _____ Blood in the urine

44. _____ Production of abnormally large amounts of urine

45. _____ Scant amount of urine (less than 500 mL in 24 hours)

46. _____ Frequent urination at night

47. _____ An artificial opening between the ureter and the abdomen

A. Polyuria

B. Ureterostomy

C. Oliguria

D. Dysuria

E. Hematuria

F. Nocturia

FILL IN THE BLANKS

48. When do most people usually void during the day? (Normal voiding routine)
   a. _____
   b. _____
   c. _____

49. Explain the two basic methods of bladder training.
   a. _____
   b. _____

Copyright © 2018 Elsevier Canada, a division of Reed Elsevier Canada, Ltd.

The next five fill-in-the-blank exercises (questions 50 through 54) each describe a common urinary problem. Identify the problem and list the causes of each problem.

50. Painful or difficult urination is called _____.

    Causes:

    a. _____

    b. _____

    c. _____

51. Blood in the urine is called _____.

    Causes:

    a. _____

    b. _____

    c. _____

52. Frequent urination at night is called _____.

    Causes:

    a. _____

    b. _____

    c. _____

53. Scant amount of urine (less than 500 mL in 24 hours) is called _____.

    Causes:

    a. _____

    b. _____

    c. _____

    d. _____

    e. _____

54. Production of abnormally large amounts of urine is called _____.

    a. _____

    b. _____

    c. _____

    d. _____

55. A ureterostomy is _____
    _____

LABELLING

Answer questions 57 through 59 using the following illustration.

56. Draw an arrow to show the direction to clean the catheter.

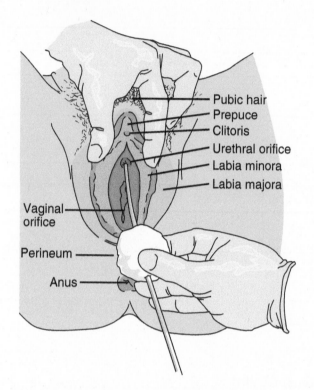

Pubic hair
Prepuce
Clitoris
Urethral orifice
Labia minora
Labia majora
Vaginal orifice
Perineum
Anus

List observations you make that need to be reported to the nurse when caring for a person with an in-dwelling catheter.

a. _____

b. _____

c. _____

d. _____

57. Name the parts of the urinary drainage system indicated.

a. _____

b. _____

c. _____

d. _____

e. _____

58. Why is the tubing coiled on the bed?

_____

_____

59. Why is the catheter taped to the man's abdomen?

_____

_____

Copyright © 2018 Elsevier Canada, a division of Reed Elsevier Canada, Ltd.

CROSSWORD

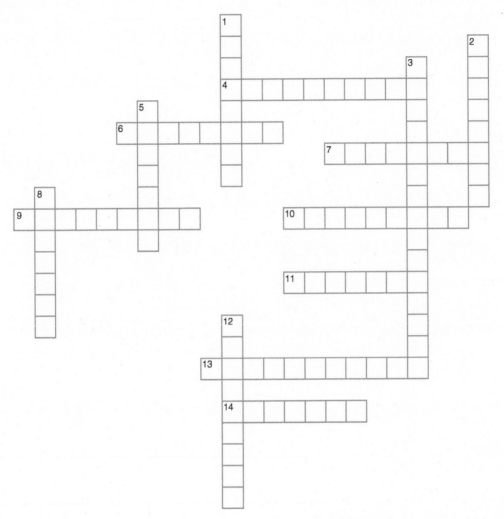

Across

4. Sugar in the urine

6. Production of abnormally large amounts of urine

7. Tube used to drain or inject fluid through a body opening

9. Voiding at frequent intervals

10. Blood in the urine

11. Painful or difficult urination

13. Process of emptying urine from the bladder; urination or voiding

14. A compound that appears in the urine because of rapid breakdown of fat for energy; ketone body.

Down

1. Scant amount of urine; usually less than 500 mL in 24 hours

2. Frequent urination at night

3. Process of inserting a catheter

5. Urination or micturition

8. Need to void immediately

12. Process of emptying urine from bladder; micturition or voiding

Copyright © 2018 Elsevier Canada, a division of Reed Elsevier Canada, Ltd.

Bowel Elimination

TRUE OR FALSE

Circle T for true, or circle F for false.

1. **T** **F** Feces move through the intestine by a process called *defecation*.

2. **T** **F** Constipation is a condition in which bowel movements are less frequent than usual.

3. **T** **F** Liquid feces seeping from the anus is not a sign of fecal impaction.

4. **T** **F** Fewer than 10 wet diapers per day from an infant may indicate dehydration.

5. **T** **F** Enemas can be dangerous.

6. **T** **F** A support worker is allowed to insert rectal tubes to relieve flatulence.

7. **T** **F** A stoma is painful when touched.

8. **T** **F** A client with an ostomy pouch can wear normal clothes.

9. **T** **F** When internal bleeding is suspected, feces are checked for blood.

10. **T** **F** A commercial enema stimulates and distends the rectum.

11. **T** **F** Feces become hard and dry when fluid intake is poor.

12. **T** **F** The support worker may help to prevent fecal incontinence by promptly responding to all requests for help using the bathroom, bedpan, or commode.

13. **T** **F** One of two goals of bowel training is to develop a regular pattern of elimination, thus preventing fecal impaction, constipation, and fecal incontinence.

14. **T** **F** When you are helping a client with bowel training, the client is usually encouraged to use the toilet, commode, or bedpan before a meal.

15. **T** **F** A suppository is used to stimulate defecation when bowel training is being done.

16. **T** **F** Giving an enema is a controlled act.

17. **T** **F** Enemas may be ordered by the physician to prepare the client for certain X-ray procedures.

18. **T** **F** The volume of saline enema varies according to a child's size and age.

Copyright © 2018 Elsevier Canada, a division of Reed Elsevier Canada, Ltd.

19. **T**   **F**   The purpose of an ostomy pouch is to collect feces and flatus.

20. **T**   **F**   An ostomy bag is changed every day and whenever it leaks.

21. **T**   **F**   An ostomy pouch can be removed and changed when peristalsis is less active. The best time is usually after breakfast.

22. **T**   **F**   Feces from an ileostomy is especially irritating to the skin because the small intestine contains digestive juices that are very irritating.

23. **T**   **F**   Occult blood is bright red blood that can be easily observed in the stool.

MULTIPLE RESPONSE

From the list below, choose all of the correct answers.

24. What should you observe and report when a client has a bowel movement?
    A.   Abnormalities in colour
    B.   Abnormalities in amount
    C.   Abnormalities in consistency
    D.   Abnormalities in odour
    E.   Abnormalities in shape
    F.   Abnormalities in size
    G.   Abnormalities in frequency
    H.   Complaints of pain

25. What are some signs of fecal impaction?
    A.   Abdominal discomfort and swelling
    B.   Cramping
    C.   A feeling of fullness or pain in the rectum
    D.   Nausea or vomiting
    E.   Fever
    F.   Increased need or decreased ability to urinate
    G.   Liquid feces seeping from the anus
    H.   Regular bowel movements

26. What are common causes of constipation?
    A.   A high-fibre diet
    B.   Ignoring the urge to defecate
    C.   Decreased fluid intake
    D.   Activity
    E.   Medications
    F.   Aging
    G.   Certain diseases

27. Which of the following comfort and safety measures can the support worker use when assisting a client with fecal elimination?
    A.   Assist the client to the toilet or commode, or provide the bedpan, as soon as requested.
    B.   Provide for privacy (ask visitors to leave the room, close doors, pull privacy curtains, and close window curtains, blinds, or shades).
    C.   Make sure the bedpan is cold.
    D.   Position the client in a side-lying position.
    E.   Allow enough time for defecation. Do not rush the client.
    F.   Place the call bell and toilet tissue within reach.
    G.   Leave the room if the client is weak or unsteady.
    H.   Provide oral care.
    I.   Dispose of stool promptly.
    J.   Assist the client with hand hygiene after elimination.

28. What symptoms may occur if flatulence is not relieved?
    A.   Abdominal cramping or pain
    B.   Shortness of breath
    C.   Decreased level of consciousness
    D.   Swollen abdomen, or "bloating"

29. Which of the following are reasons that enemas are given?
    A.   To remove feces
    B.   To relieve constipation or fecal impaction
    C.   To encourage weight loss
    D.   To clean the bowel of feces before certain surgeries or X-ray procedures
    E.   To relieve flatulence and intestinal distension

Copyright © 2018 Elsevier Canada, a division of Reed Elsevier Canada, Ltd.

30. How can odour associated with an ostomy pouch be prevented?
    A. By providing good hygiene
    B. Instructing the client to cover it with a plastic bag
    C. By encouraging the client to avoid gas-forming foods
    D. By putting deodorants into the pouch, according to the care plan

MULTIPLE CHOICE

Circle the correct answer.

31. Which of the following will not assist fecal elimination?
    A. Drinking a hot beverage
    B. Using a bedside commode in a semiprivate room
    C. Taking a walk
    D. Reading a book or newspaper

32. Which of these foods would be most likely to stimulate fecal elimination?
    A. Pudding and gelatin
    B. Whole-grain cereals and fruit
    C. Meat and fish
    D. Pretzels and potato chips

33. Mr. Lane, 85, usually has a bowel movement after breakfast. About 45 minutes after having a bowel movement, he wants to go to the bathroom again. The most likely reason for this is:
    A. Older adults lose control over defecation.
    B. Complete emptying of the rectum does not always occur with older adults.
    C. He may have a tumour or other disorder.
    D. He is concerned about becoming constipated.

34. Which of these may kill normal flora in the intestine?
    A. Antibiotics
    B. Laxatives
    C. Pain medications
    D. Enemas

35. What instruction will the nurse likely give if a client has diarrhea?
    A. Withhold all fluids.
    B. Give the client plenty to drink.
    C. Encourage the client to eat as little as possible.
    D. Give the client foods with plenty of fibre.

36. What would be an effective nursing action to relieve flatulence?
    A. Giving an enema
    B. Making sure the diet is high in vegetables
    C. Having the client lie flat in bed
    D. Ambulating the client or placing the client in the side-lying position

37. When the nurse inserts a suppository to stimulate defecation, how soon would you expect results?
    A. In about 30 minutes
    B. Immediately
    C. In 2 to 3 hours
    D. In the morning

38. Which position is best when giving an enema?
    A. Sims' position
    B. Right position
    C. Semi-Fowler's position
    D. Prone position

39. Which of the following statements about stool specimens is correct?
    A. Stool specimens are best obtained at the end of the day.
    B. Urine will contaminate the stool specimen.
    C. Stool specimens should be sent to the lab by the end of each shift.
    D. Stool specimens that contain blood have been contaminated and should not be accepted.

Copyright © 2018 Elsevier Canada, a division of Reed Elsevier Canada, Ltd.

40. You should wear gloves when testing a stool for occult blood to:
    A. Prevent contact with body fluids and substances
    B. Prevent contaminating the specimen
    C. Maintain a sterile specimen
    D. Prevent contact with chemicals used in the test

41. The term *melena* describes stool that:
    A. Is black and tarry
    B. Contains unseen blood
    C. Hard and pebble-shaped
    D. Contains visible parasites

42. What is the purpose of a rectal tube?
    A. Relief of constipation
    B. Treatment of fecal impaction
    C. Prevention of diarrhea
    D. Relief of flatulence and distension

43. What is the consistency of the stool if a colostomy is near the end of the large intestine?
    A. Liquid
    B. Soft
    C. Formed
    D. Hard and dry

44. Which of these methods would help to prevent skin breakdown around the stoma?
    A. Clean with alcohol wipes.
    B. Use an antiseptic lotion or petroleum jelly on the skin.
    C. Clean the area with water and mild soap as directed by the nurse.
    D. Wipe with tissues until clean.

MATCHING

Match each of the corresponding factors that can cause the stool to change colours to the correct colour.

45. _____ Bleeding in the stomach

46. _____ Bleeding in the lower colon or rectum; also, beets

47. _____ A diet high in green vegetables

A. Green

B. Black

C. Red

Copyright © 2018 Elsevier Canada, a division of Reed Elsevier Canada, Ltd.

Match each definition to the correct word.

48. _____ Semi-solid mass of waste products in the colon

49. _____ Introduction of fluid into the rectum and lower colon

50. _____ Artificial opening between the ileum and abdomen

51. _____ Bowel movement

52. _____ Alternating contraction and relaxation of intestinal muscles

53. _____ Surgical creation of an artificial opening

54. _____ Cone-shaped medication that is inserted into a body opening

55. _____ Gas or air in the stomach or intestines

56. _____ Feces that have been excreted

57. _____ Frequent passage of liquid stools

58. _____ Partially digested food and fluids that pass from the stomach to the small intestine

59. _____ The opening of a colostomy or ileostomy

A. Defecation

B. Suppository

C. Diarrhea

D. Peristalsis

E. Feces

F. Ostomy

G. Enema

H. Chyme

I. Flatus

J. Stoma

K. Stool

L. Ileostomy

FILL IN THE BLANKS

60. What effect does normal bacterial action in the large intestine have on the stool? _____
_____

61. What are the risks if you do not give good skin care to a client who has diarrhea?

   a. _____

   b. _____

   c. _____

62. How would you mix the solution for a saline enema? _____
_____

63. How does a commercial enema, which contains only 120 mL of solution, stimulate defecation? _____
_____

64. When you are giving "enemas until clear," how will you know that you have given enough? _____
_____

Copyright © 2018 Elsevier Canada, a division of Reed Elsevier Canada, Ltd.

65. How warm is the solution in a cleansing enema? _____

66. Only a _____ enema may be given to children.

67. What instructions should you give to a client who is going to expel an enema in the toilet? _____
_____

68. What will happen if you release pressure on a commercial enema container while giving an enema?
_____

69. What is the purpose of an ostomy pouch? _____

70. You should empty or open an ostomy pouch when _____ or when the
bag _____.

71. An ostomy bag is changed every _____ days.

72. An ostomy pouch can be removed and changed when peristalsis is less active. The best time is usually
_____.

73. Why are certain stool specimens taken directly to the laboratory? _____
_____

Refer to the figure when answering Questions 74–76:

74. a. How high above the anus should the bag hang? _____

   b. How high above the mattress should bag hang? _____

75. How far should the tube be inserted into the rectum? _____

76. Identify the position of the person. _____
_____

Copyright © 2018 Elsevier Canada, a division of Reed Elsevier Canada, Ltd.

WORD SEARCH

Write the correct word next to each definition below. Then find those words in the Word Search and circle or highlight them in the puzzle.

77. _____ Semi-solid mass of waste products in the colon

78. _____ Introduction of fluid into the rectum and lower colon

79. _____ Artificial opening between the ileum and abdomen

80. _____ Bowel movement

81. _____ Alternating contraction and relaxation of intestinal muscles

82. _____ Surgical creation of an artificial opening

83. _____ Cone-shaped medication that is inserted into a body opening

84. _____ Gas or air in the stomach or intestines

85. _____ Feces that have been excreted

86. _____ Frequent passage of liquid stools

87. _____Partially digested food and fluids that pass from the stomach to the small intestine

88. _____ The opening of a colostomy or ileostomy

I	B	O	W	E	A	E	L	I	M	I	N	A	T	I	O	N	S
N	S	U	N	N	Y	M	A	F	I	N	D	R	O	N	T	O	T
C	U	Q	O	L	I	T	E	E	N	L	E	A	P	F	R	O	U
O	P	U	S	T	L	C	T	N	D	A	F	S	L	L	O	L	D
N	P	A	T	G	E	N	T	L	E	M	E	K	A	A	L	A	Y
T	O	L	O	S	O	L	I	F	E	M	C	I	S	T	O	M	A
I	S	I	O	G	S	L	A	N	U	S	A	N	A	U	T	W	A
N	I	T	L	E	T	P	E	R	I	S	T	A	L	S	I	S	R
E	T	Y	O	F	O	D	R	Y	P	R	I	V	C	C	Y	M	D
N	O	S	T	O	M	Y	T	I	N	L	O	V	E	H	A	H	N
C	R	O	T	O	Y	A	K	I	N	O	N	E	S	S	Y	O	O
E	Y	L	I	F	E	D	I	A	R	R	H	E	A	S	L	M	W
B	O	W	E	L	T	R	A	I	N	I	N	G	P	L	A	N	E

Copyright © 2018 Elsevier Canada, a division of Reed Elsevier Canada, Ltd.

Beds and Bed Making

TRUE OR FALSE

Circle T for true, or circle F for false.

1. **T   F** In long-term care, an open bed is made because most clients are out of bed all day.

2. **T   F** Clients in long-term care facilities may use their own linens.

3. **T   F** If a client receiving home care refuses to have his linens changed, you should follow the client's wishes.

4. **T   F** The space between the mattress and crib sides should be no more than 5 cm (2 in.).

5. **T   F** A surgical bed is made by fan-folding the linens to the side of the bed closest to the door.

6. **T   F** Shaking bed linens spreads microbes.

7. **T   F** Making one side of the bed before going to the other saves the support worker time and energy.

MULTIPLE RESPONSE

From the list below, choose all of the correct answers.

8. Which bed-making steps follow Standard Practices?
   A. Hold linens away from your body.
   B. Roll up the soiled linen away from you.
   C. Wear gloves when handling soiled linen.
   D. Very soiled linens should be placed on the floor to avoid further contamination.

9. When you are making an occupied bed, which of the following are concerns you should have about the client in the bed?
   A. Ensure the client is in good body alignment.
   B. Know about restrictions or limitations concerning the client's movement or positioning.
   C. Ensure the garbage is removed from the room.
   D. Each step of the procedure should be explained to the client.

Copyright © 2018 Elsevier Canada, a division of Reed Elsevier Canada, Ltd.

10. Identify the correct basic bed positions:
    A. Fowler's position
    B. Reverse Fowler's position
    C. Trendelenburg position
    D. Reverse Trendelenburg position
    E. Semi-Trendelenburg position
    F. Semi-Fowler's position
    G. Flat

MULTIPLE CHOICE

Circle the correct answer.

11. When changing bed linens, when should you wear gloves?
    A. If you have not performed hand hygiene.
    B. When linens are soiled with blood, body fluids, or body secretions or excretions
    C. When you are handling the clean linens
    D. Before the client has had a bath

12. Which statement is true when you are making an occupied bed?
    A. Remove all soiled linens before starting.
    B. Position the client on the side of the bed opposite to the side you are making.
    C. The top linens are folded so that a client can be transferred from a stretcher to the bed easily.
    D. If used, the clean incontinence pad is placed directly onto the mattress.

13. Why do you raise the level of the bed when you are changing linens?
    A. So that you can use good body mechanics to prevent injury
    B. To prevent injury to the client in bed
    C. To allow space under the bed for cleaning
    D. So that you can keep the client in good body alignment

14. The high-Fowler's position is used in order to:
    A. Decrease the client's rate of breathing
    B. Reduce the risk of choking while eating
    C. Promote the client's renal function
    D. Reduce the client's ankle swelling

15. An alternating pressure mattress:
    A. Cannot be placed in a high-Fowler's position.
    B. Requires that all sheets be tightly tucked under the mattress.
    C. Requires the use of an incontinence pad at all times.
    D. Is used for clients who are prone to skin breakdown.

MATCHING

Match each term with the correct statement.

16. _____ Closed bed

17. _____ Open bed

18. _____ Occupied bed

19. _____ Hospital bed

20. _____ Bottom sheet

A. Top linens are folded for transferring the client to or from a stretcher

B. Can be raised horizontally to give care

C. A bed made with the client in it

D. Top linens are pulled up and the bedspread is pulled neatly over the pillow

E. Must be wrinkle free to prevent skin irritation

Copyright © 2018 Elsevier Canada, a division of Reed Elsevier Canada, Ltd.

FILL IN THE BLANKS

21. Why is an incontinence pad used on the bed? _____

22. What is the disadvantage of using an incontinence pad? _____
    _____

23. When making an occupied bed, the client should be covered with a bath blanket to provide _____
    _____ and _____.

24. What are the safety rules about using bumper pads on a crib?

    a. _____
    b. _____
    c. _____
    d. _____

LABELLING

25. Arrange in order the steps used to make a mitred corner, by writing the letters "A" through "D" on
    the line below.

_____

Copyright © 2018 Elsevier Canada, a division of Reed Elsevier Canada, Ltd.

Mental Health Disorders

TRUE OR FALSE

Circle T for true, or circle F for false.

1. T F A mental health disorder can affect all dimensions of a person's life.

2. T F Depressive disorders are usually mild in nature.

3. T F The onset of most mental health disorders occurs in mid- to late-life.

4. T F Anxiety disorders are the least common of all mental health issues.

5. T F Communication is important when caring for persons with mental health disorders.

6. T F Panic disorders are more common in women.

7. T F A panic attack occurs suddenly with no obvious reason.

8. T F When a panic attack occurs, the client may experience racing heart and even chest pain.

9. T F A *phobia* involves intense fear of an object or situation.

10. T F Selective mutism is an inability or extreme reluctance to speak in certain social situations.

11. T F In the manic phase of bipolar disorder, the person feels depressed and worthless.

12. T F Depression in the older adult is rarely overlooked.

13. T F Major depression can occur at any age.

14. T F *Psychosis* is a mental disorder in which the perception of reality is impaired.

15. T F *Delusion* is the uncontrollable urge to perform an act.

16. T F The term *hallucination* is another word for sleepwalking.

17. T F Schizophrenia affects one's ability to function in all aspects of life.

18. T F Someone who has schizophrenia has a split personality.

Copyright © 2018 Elsevier Canada, a division of Reed Elsevier Canada, Ltd.

19. **T   F**   Without treatment, the person who has schizophrenia has problems knowing what is real and what is not.

20. **T   F**   People with depression might have as a symptom the belief that others are betraying them.

21. **T   F**   A *compulsion* is an unwillingness to accept reality.

22. **T   F**   An *obsession* is resentfulness toward others.

23. **T   F**   People fixated with the idea that germs are on their hands will often wash their hands repeatedly.

24. **T   F**   If a person believes he or she is the prime minister of Canada, that person is having a delusion of grandeur.

25. **T   F**   Bipolar affective disorders are easy to diagnose in children.

26. **T   F**   An older client with fatigue, slow or unreliable memory, agitation, and thoughts of death may be suffering from depression.

27. **T   F**   A client with anorexia nervosa craves food; after eating, the person induces vomiting.

28. **T   F**   Some people who are bulimic take diuretics to lose weight.

29. **T   F**   A client with schizophrenia may experience delusions and hallucinations.

30. **T   F**   A person with anxiety experiences vague, uneasy feelings and feels a sense of danger or harm.

31. **T   F**   To support a client with a disruptive, impulse-control, and conduct disorder, you should try to hug the client.

32. **T   F**   For optimal mental health functioning, teenagers should get 5 to 6 hours of sleep each night.

MULTIPLE RESPONSE

From the list below, choose all of the correct answers.

33. What are some of the causes of mental health disorders?
    A. Biological factors
    B. Extreme intelligence
    C. Childhood trauma or conflict
    D. Social and cultural factors (e.g., poverty, discrimination, social isolation)
    E. Stressful life events (e.g., death of a loved one, divorce)
    F. Poor physical health or disability

34. The various forms of psychotherapy include:
    A. Psychoanalysis
    B. Behaviour therapy
    C. Group therapy
    D. Diet therapy
    E. Family therapy

35. A person suffering from schizophrenia may exhibit the following behaviours:
    A. Psychosis
    B. Delusions
    C. Increased need for sleeping
    D. Hallucinations
    E. Paranoia

Copyright © 2018 Elsevier Canada, a division of Reed Elsevier Canada, Ltd.

36. Signs and symptoms of depression include:
    A. Bloating and flatulence
    B. Feeling sad, "blue," or hopeless
    C. Itchy skin and hives
    D. Irritability
    E. Reduced interest in almost all activities
    F. Significant weight gain or loss, without dieting
    G. Insomnia or too much sleep
    H. Too much or too little motor activity
    I. Fatigue or loss of energy
    J. Feelings of worthlessness or guilt
    K. Strong desire to eat a nonfood substance
    L. Increased ability to concentrate or think
    M. Difficulties making decisions
    N. Recurrent thoughts of death

37. Which of these factors may contribute to a mental health disorder?
    A. Poor physical health and lifestyle
    B. Loving and satisfying relationships
    C. Inability to cope with stressful life events
    D. Family members with a mental health disorder
    E. Ability to handle challenging situations
    F. Traumatic past life experiences

38. Which are common risk factors for suicidal intent in an older adult?
    A. Loss of independence
    B. Ability to adapt to change
    C. Unable to manage finances without assistance
    D. Ability to obtain groceries
    E. Extreme losses in friends and family
    F. Chronic pain that interferes with sleep

MULTIPLE CHOICE

Circle the correct answer.

39. An acquired brain injury (ABI) is defined as:
    A. Inability to cope with stress and anxiety
    B. The effects from long-term excessive alcohol abuse
    C. Any lasting traumatic emotional experience
    D. Any type of sudden injury that causes brain damage

40. Which of the following is an example of an unhealthy coping response to stress?
    A. Going for a walk
    B. Exercising
    C. Chain smoking
    D. Having a piece of cake with a meal

41. An older adult may not be diagnosed with depression because:
    A. It rarely occurs in an older adult
    B. Treatment of physical problems is more important in an older adult
    C. The older person may be thought to have dementia
    D. Depression in older adults is usually mild and does not require treatment

42. Which of these would be present in someone with delusions of persecution?
    A. Seeing, hearing, or feeling something that is not there
    B. Not sleeping or taking time to tend to self-care needs
    C. Believing that one is mistreated, abused, or harassed
    D. Having poor judgement and morals and lacking ethics

43. When a person has anorexia nervosa, which of these behaviours is likely to be displayed?
    A. Dieting even though the person becomes emaciated
    B. Withdrawing from the world and showing no interest in others
    C. Regressing to the behaviour of a younger child
    D. Having delusions or hallucinations

44. Which of these substances can be abused?
    A. Legal drugs
    B. Illegal drugs
    C. Alcohol
    D. All of the above

Copyright © 2018 Elsevier Canada, a division of Reed Elsevier Canada, Ltd.

45. Which of the following statements about post-traumatic stress disorder (PTSD) is true?
    A. People with PTSD will often voluntarily share their experiences.
    B. PTSD occurs only in adults.
    C. Survivors with PTSD will most likely improve without counselling.
    D. PTSD is a trauma- or stress-related disorder.

46. What is the best response to use when caring for a client who is depressed?
    A. "Let me tell you a funny story."
    B. "You seem down today."
    C. "Cheer up and don't look so sad."
    D. "Don't worry; everything will be all right."

47. When caring for a client who has a substance-related and addictive disorder, you should:
    A. Confront the client in a professional manner if you suspect the client is abusing alcohol.
    B. Discuss suspicions of alcohol abuse only with your supervisor.
    C. Say nothing to anybody to respect the client's right to confidentiality.
    D. Locate the alcohol and discretely pour it down the drain.

48. Mr. Wong becomes very angry and states that someone has been in his room and has taken his razor. He is swearing and yelling at the staff. Your best response is:
    A. "I don't blame you for being angry."
    B. "That doesn't make any sense. I don't know who would want your razor."
    C. "This happens all the time" and begin to look in his bedside unit.
    D. "This is very upsetting. Can you show me where you usually keep your razor?"

49. Which statement in regard to suicide is correct?
    A. Suicidal intent is a sign of a serious physical health problem.
    B. More women die by suicide than men.
    C. Men use less violent means than women to die by suicide.
    D. Suicide is a common cause of death among adolescents.

50. You suspect a client has suicidal intent. What should you do?
    A. Quietly collect all the client's pills and place them in a paper bag.
    B. Stay with the client but inform your supervisor immediately.
    C. Tell the person that "everyone has those thoughts."
    D. Recommend that the client take another anxiety pill with her tea.

FILL IN THE BLANKS

51. An obsession is _____.

52. A compulsion is _____.

53. Why does a person act on an obsessive idea?
    _____

54. If a person believes he or she is the prime minister of Canada, what type of false belief is present? _____

55. An older person has the following symptoms: fatigue, slow or unreliable memory, agitation, and thoughts of death. It may be that he or she is suffering from _____.

56. A person with _____ craves food. After eating, the person induces
    _____

57. Why does a person with bulimia take diuretics?
    _____

58. What do the following statements describe?
    - Thinking and behaviour are disturbed
    - Delusions and hallucinations are present
    - The individual has difficulty relating to others and the world

    _____

59. What do the following statements describe?
    - The individual has vague, uneasy feelings
    - The person feels a sense of danger or harm
    - Occurs in response to stress
    - The person is unaware of the source of the uneasy feeling

    _____

60. What do the following statements describe?
    - The person may have extreme mood swings
    - At times, the person may feel very sad, lonely, worthless
    - Tends to run in families
    - At times, the person may have much energy and be excited

    _____

61. What do the following statements describe?
    - Abusive
    - Paranoid
    - Distrusts others
    - Irresponsible

    _____

Copyright © 2018 Elsevier Canada, a division of Reed Elsevier Canada, Ltd.

Disorientation, Delirium, and Dementia

TRUE OR FALSE

Circle T for true, or circle F for false.

1. **T** **F** Never tell a disoriented client the date and time.

2. **T** **F** When caring for disoriented clients, you should provide newspapers and magazines and access to television and radio.

3. **T** **F** It is all right to rearrange the furniture or belongings of a disoriented client.

4. **T** **F** Delirium is a permanent state of mental disorientation.

5. **T** **F** Delirium is an emergency.

6. **T** **F** Repetitive behaviours that are harmless may cause no problems to the client.

7. **T** **F** People with Alzheimer's disease can control their behaviours of forgetfulness, incontinence, agitation, or rudeness if they are shown how.

8. **T** **F** Alzheimer's disease progresses slowly at a predictable rate in all people.

9. **T** **F** It is important to reason with a patient who is cognitively impaired as a first step when the client is behaving in an aggressive manner.

10. **T** **F** Individuals who have a cognitive impairment are not likely to be physically abused.

11. **T** **F** Always approach a cognitively impaired client in an assertive and controlling manner.

12. **T** **F** Delirium is the same as dementia.

13. **T** **F** The average age of people with Alzheimer's disease and related dementias is 42 years.

14. **T   F**   A client with dementia is in danger of having accidents because the client does not recognize safety hazards.

15. **T   F**   A *catastrophic reaction* refers to a mild response to a perceived danger.

16. **T   F**   *Hoarding* is intentionally obtaining information about a client.

17. **T   F**   When caring for a disoriented client, face the client and speak clearly and slowly.

18. **T   F**   You should maintain a disoriented client's routine by following a schedule for meals, bathing, exercise, TV, and other activities.

19. **T   F**   Cueing at mealtime is an important way to assist a client who has middle-stage dementia.

20. **T   F**   The *sandwich generation* refers to adult children who care for their own children and their parents.

21. **T   F**   *Sundowning* refers to the way daylight can cause an anxiety reaction in some clients.

22. **T   F**   A disoriented client can become more disoriented if not wearing glasses.

MULTIPLE RESPONSE

From the list below, choose all of the correct answers.

23. Early warning signs of dementia may include:
    A.   Memory loss that affects daily activities
    B.   Disorientation
    C.   Problems finding the right words or following conversations
    D.   Poor judgement
    E.   Urinary urgency
    F.   Problems with common tasks
    G.   Changes in mood, behaviour, or personality
    H.   Loss of interest in activities or hobbies

24. Some of the *behaviours* associated with early-stage dementia include:
    A.   Increase in spontaneity—more outgoing or interested in things
    B.   Problems finishing thoughts, following directions, and remembering names
    C.   Poor judgement
    D.   Blaming others for mistakes, forgetfulness, and other problems
    E.   Irritability or defensiveness
    F.   Problems performing everyday tasks

25. Ways that caregivers can help to calm a person with dementia who screams include:
    A.   Providing a calm, quiet setting
    B.   Using touch to calm the client
    C.   Playing soft music
    D.   Discouraging the client from wearing hearing aids to reduce noise
    E.   Having a family member or favourite caregiver comfort and calm the client

26. What should you do when a client with Alzheimer's disease fondles her genital area?
    A.   Check to see if the client is wet or soiled.
    B.   Provide for privacy and safety for the client.
    C.   Notify your supervisor if this is a frequent behaviour
    D.   Ask the client's family to bring in sex magazines so the client can look at them

Copyright © 2018 Elsevier Canada, a division of Reed Elsevier Canada, Ltd.

27. What are some reasons a family may decide to place a person with Alzheimer's disease in a long-term care facility?
    A. Clients with Alzheimer's disease are not allowed to be in a private home.
    B. Family members cannot meet the person's needs.
    C. Family members have their own health problems.
    D. The person's behaviours present a danger to herself or to others.

MULTIPLE CHOICE

Circle the correct answer.

28. How can you maintain the day–night cycle for a disoriented client?
    A. Keep the room well lit all day and at night
    B. Keep the curtains closed in the client's room all day
    C. Encourage the person to wear regular clothes during the day, not sleepwear
    D. Do not allow the client to be toileted during the night

29. Which statement is true concerning clients with Alzheimer's disease and sundowning?
    A. The client may be frightened by poor light or shadows.
    B. Sundowning occurs only on clear nights when the moon is visible.
    C. The client can be talked out of his fears.
    D. There is no treatment for sundowning.

30. Which of the following actions may increase a client's disorientation?
    A. Stating your name and showing your name tag
    B. Giving the client very detailed instructions prior to performing a procedure
    C. Calling the client by name each time you are in contact with him
    D. Encouraging the client to wear his glasses and hearing aid if needed

31. Which of these measures is helpful when a client with Alzheimer's disease is agitated?
    A. Approach the client in a slow, unhurried manner.
    B. Turn the volume of the TV up to get the client's attention.
    C. Gently begin massaging the client's back.
    D. Place the client in a darkened room and shut the door.

32. What should you do if the client repeatedly tries to go outside and wander?
    A. Make sure the client receives medication to calm him or her down.
    B. Restrain the client to prevent wandering.
    C. If allowed, escort the client outside and stay with him or her.
    D. Tell the client he or she is not allowed outside.

33. How can you incorporate principles of validation therapy when caring for a client who thinks that "kitty cats" are in her closet?
    A. Ask her to describe the cats
    B. Distract her by showing her pictures on her dresser
    C. Tell her that there are no cats in that facility
    D. Ask her if she is hungry

34. Vascular dementia is:
    A. The least common form of dementia
    B. Is also called Creutzfeldt-Jakob disease
    C. Is the result of a series of strokes
    D. Is caused by a lack of Vitamin D in the diet

35. A broad term describing a progressive deterioration of intellectual function is:
    A. Dementia
    B. Mental health disorder
    C. Senility
    D. Schizophrenia

Copyright © 2018 Elsevier Canada, a division of Reed Elsevier Canada, Ltd.

36. Which of the following is a reversible form of dementia?
    A. Parkinson's disease
    B. Brain tumour
    C. Normal pressure hydrocephalus
    D. Multiple sclerosis

37. Pseudo-dementia occurs when:
    A. Pathogens destroy nerve cells in the brain
    B. Thiamine is in high levels in the body
    C. The cells multiply, forming a brain tumour
    D. When severe depression causes cognitive changes, mimicking dementia

38. What is a classic sign of Alzheimer's disease?
    A. Problems finding one's car keys
    B. Repeatedly saying the same statement
    C. Engaging in reckless behaviour
    D. Forgetting how to perform long division

39. What is apraxia?
    A. A sudden increase in cursing or swearing
    B. Temporary mental disorientation
    C. The loss of being able to perform learned skills
    D. A sudden loss of hair

40. Apathy can be described as:
    A. Extreme mood swings within a short time period
    B. A defence mechanism when communicating
    C. An absence of emotional feeling
    D. A display of increased anxiety

MATCHING

Match the area of concern for people with dementia with its correct care strategy.

41. _____ Follow facility policy for locking doors and windows.

42. _____ Provide plastic eating and drinking utensils.

43. _____ Tell the client that you will provide protection from harm.

44. _____ Give consistent responses.

45. _____ Provide for the client's food and fluid needs.

46. _____ Play music and show movies from the client's past.

47. _____ Make sure the client has eaten, because hunger can increase restlessness.

A. Loss of short-term memory

B. Forgetting a person, place, or time

C. Risk for injury

D. Wandering

E. Sundowning

F. Hallucinations and delusions

G. Reduced ability to meet one's own basic needs

Copyright © 2018 Elsevier Canada, a division of Reed Elsevier Canada, Ltd.

Match the area of concern for people with dementia with a strategy to give care to address that concern.

48. _____Try bathing the client when he or she is calm.

49. _____Make sure the client wears an ID bracelet at all times.

50. _____Approach the client in a calm, quiet manner.

51. _____Provide a quiet and calm eating environment. Cue chewing behaviours as needed.

52. _____Ensure the client's eyeglasses and hearing aids are clean and in good repair. Keep area well lit and play soft music.

53. _____Keep a calendar and clock where the client can see them.

A. Disorientation to place and time

B. Displays of aggressive behaviour if startled

C. Easily distracted during meals

D. Wandering

E. Hallucinations and delusions

F. Fear of personal care

FILL IN THE BLANKS

Match the signs and symptoms below with the following conditions:
A. Disorientation
B. Dementia

54. _____ Loss of ability to recognize own reflection in a mirror

55. _____ Can occur after surgery

56. _____ Anger, restlessness, depression, and irritability may occur

57. _____ May be caused by losses of hearing and sight

58. _____ Progressive loss of cognitive and social functions

Place the letter of the stage of dementia next to the symptom that best describes it:
A. Stage 1
B. Stage 2
C. Stage 3

59. _____ Restlessness that increases during evening hours

60. _____ Cannot walk or sit

Copyright © 2018 Elsevier Canada, a division of Reed Elsevier Canada, Ltd.

61. _____ Less outgoing and less interested in things

62. _____ Forgets recent events

63. _____ Does not recognize family members

64. _____ May say the same thing over and over again

65. _____ Cannot tell the difference between hot and cold

66. _____ Totally incontinent of urine and feces

67. _____ Disoriented to time and place

68. _____ Cannot communicate

69. _____ Has difficulty following directions

70. Delirium is common in _____ with _____ illnesses.

71. The risk of Alzheimer's disease increases after the age of _____.

72. Describe each of the following problems that occur with dementia or the behaviour that is displayed with the problem.

   a. Catastrophic reactions _____

   _____

   b. Agitation and restlessness _____

   _____

   c. Aggression and combativeness _____

   _____

   d. Screaming _____

   _____

   e. Abnormal sexual behaviour _____

   _____

   f. Repetitive behaviours _____

   _____

73. What actions by a caregiver can cause agitation and restlessness?

   _____

74. How can you help someone with Alzheimer's disease who displays abnormal sexual behaviour?

_____

_____

75. What are reasons why sundowning may occur in a person with Alzheimer's disease?

   a. _____

   b. _____

   c. _____

76. What response may occur if a person with Alzheimer's disease receives too many stimuli at one time?

_____

77. Complete these statements that relate to providing care for a confused client.

   a. Face the person and _____.

   b. Explain what _____.

   c. Give short, simple _____.

   d. Keep calendars and clocks with _____.

   e. Allow the person to place _____.

   f. Ask _____ questions. Allow enough time _____

   _____.

   g. Maintain _____ atmosphere.

78. Why are locks placed at the top or bottom of a door to prevent wandering?

_____

79. Why is it ineffective to argue or try to reason with a person with Alzheimer's disease?

_____

Copyright © 2018 Elsevier Canada, a division of Reed Elsevier Canada, Ltd.

Common Diseases and Conditions

TRUE OR FALSE

Circle T for true, or circle F for false.

1. T F People who have osteoarthritis experience joint stiffness with activity and range-of-motion exercises.

2. T F Rheumatoid arthritis affects only the large weight-bearing joints.

3. T F Rheumatoid arthritis in children can affect growth and development.

4. T F Arthroplasty is done to cure arthritis.

5. T F People can help to prevent osteoporosis by taking calcium supplements and having a regular exercise program.

6. T F When turning and repositioning a client with osteoporosis, you should move him or her quickly to prevent fractures.

7. T F Osteoporosis causes the cartilage that occupies the joints of the body to deteriorate.

8. T F An infant who has a fracture may be a victim of child abuse.

9. T F Phantom limb pains can occur when a client has had an amputation.

10. T F A stroke occurs when brain cells get too much oxygen and too many nutrients.

11. T F All clients with Parkinson's disease have impaired mental function.

12. T F Multiple sclerosis is a short-term, acute disease.

13. T F A client with chronic obstructive pulmonary disease (COPD) is at risk for respiratory infections.

14. T F The use of condoms is one way to reduce the spread of tuberculosis.

Copyright © 2018 Elsevier Canada, a division of Reed Elsevier Canada, Ltd.

15. T   F   Clients with tuberculosis have an overproduction of thyroxin hormone.

16. T   F   Angina pectoris occurs when vessels narrow and the heart pumps with more force.

17. T   F   Activity will usually relieve angina pain in 3 to 15 minutes.

18. T   F   A common term for a myocardial infarction is *heart attack*.

19. T   F   The goal of cardiac rehabilitation after a myocardial infarction is to prevent another attack.

20. T   F   When a client has renal calculi, you should strain the urine.

21. T   F   When a client has persistent renal failure, only the renal system is affected.

22. T   F   You need to follow Standard Practices when disposing of vomitus.

23. T   F   A client who has human immunodeficiency virus (HIV) but has not developed acquired immune deficiency syndrome (AIDS) cannot infect others with the virus.

24. T   F   Elevated toilet seats are helpful to a client with osteoarthritis when the client has limited range of motion in the hips and knees.

25. T   F   Juvenile rheumatoid arthritis occurs in children.

26. T   F   Preventing deformities is one of the goals in treating rheumatoid arthritis.

27. T   F   When a client has osteoporosis, a fracture can occur because the bones are very brittle.

28. T   F   Shingles are caused by an allergic reaction.

29. T   F   A client with emphysema can breathe more easily if he or she is allowed to sit upright and slightly forward.

30. T   F   Exercise and physiotherapy can help a client with Parkinson's disease to improve or maintain strength, posture, balance, and mobility.

31. T   F   Repeated asthma attacks can damage the respiratory system.

32. T   F   Scabies appear as white circular patches on the lower legs and back areas.

33. T   F   The term *furuncle* is used to describe a skin tag.

34. T   F   An aneurysm is caused from the presence of excessive acid in the digestive tract.

35. T   F   Hypertension is more common among Canadians of South Asian, Aboriginal, and African descent.

36. T   F   The risk of hypertension increases if excess weight is stored around the abdomen.

37. T   F   Good skin care and regular position changes can help to prevent skin breakdown.

38. T   F   With persistent renal failure, the nephrons of the kidneys are destroyed.

39. T   F   Clients with persistent renal failure have dialysis to remove wastes and excess water from the blood.

Copyright © 2018 Elsevier Canada, a division of Reed Elsevier Canada, Ltd.

40. **T**   **F**   The most important way to prevent the spread of hepatitis is by practising Standard Practices.

41. **T**   **F**   AIDS reduces the client's ability to fight infections.

42. **T**   **F**   The use of condoms will help prevent the spread of sexually transmitted infections (STIs).

MULTIPLE RESPONSE

From the list below, choose all of the correct answers.

43. Which of the following are early warning signs of cancer?
    A. A cough that goes on for more than two days
    B. Blood in the stool
    C. Indigestion that continues more than an hour
    D. Unexplained aches and pains that go on for more than two weeks
    E. Difficulty urinating or blood in the urine
    F. Bleeding after a cut
    G. Any lump or mass
    H. A sore that does not heal
    I. A new growth on the skin
    J. Patches of skin that bleed, itch, or are red

44. What side effects of radiation therapy cause clients with cancer to have special care needs?
    A. Discomfort
    B. Nausea and vomiting
    C. Increased appetite
    D. Fatigue
    E. Diarrhea
    F. Skin breakdown

45. A child falls and has signs and symptoms of a fracture. These would include which of the following?
    A. Limb looks bent or out of position
    B. Pain
    C. Swelling
    D. Unlimited movement of limb
    E. Bruising and colour changes in the skin at the fracture site
    F. Bleeding (internal or external)

46. What treatments are used to relieve pain and stiffness in a client with osteoarthritis?
    A. Physicians may order aspirin for pain.
    B. Heat or cold applications may be ordered.
    C. Obese clients may be advised to gain weight.
    D. A low-fat, low-calorie diet may be ordered.
    E. A cane or walker may be used for support.

47. Which of the following are rules you should follow when caring for a client with a cast?
    A. Make sure to cover the cast with blankets, plastic, or other material.
    B. Turn the client as directed by the care plan.
    C. Place a wet cast on a hard surface.
    D. Support a wet cast with your palms when turning and positioning the client.
    E. Protect the client from rough cast edges.
    F. Keep a plaster cast dry.
    G. Do not allow the client to insert anything under the cast.
    H. Elevate a casted arm or leg on pillows.
    I. Have enough help when turning and repositioning the client.
    J. Position the client as directed by your supervisor and the care plan.

Copyright © 2018 Elsevier Canada, a division of Reed Elsevier Canada, Ltd.

48. When you care for a client with a hip fracture, what measures are important for you to follow?
    A. Meet basic needs if the client is confined to bed, and prevent complications of bed rest.
    B. Transfer, turn, and reposition the person as directed.
    C. Keep the operated leg adducted at all times.
    D. Encourage external rotation of the hip.
    E. Provide range-of-motion exercises as directed.
    F. Provide a straight-backed chair with armrests.
    G. Prevent the client's leg from bending at the hip.
    H. Do not let the client stand on the affected leg unless allowed by the physician.
    I. Support and elevate the leg as directed when the client is in a chair.
    J. Apply elastic stockings as directed.
    K. Remind the client that it is okay to cross the legs while seated.

49. If you are caring for a client who has had a stroke, you might observe effects such as:
    A. Hemiplegia
    B. Weakness on both sides of the body
    C. Loss of muscle control of the face
    D. Changing emotions
    E. Difficulty swallowing
    F. Dimmed vision or loss of vision
    G. Improved ability to speak or understand others
    H. Changes in sight, touch, movement, and thought
    I. Improved memory
    J. Urinary frequency, urgency, or incontinence

50. What measures would be helpful to use when you care for a client who has had a stroke?
    A. Complete all activities of daily living for the client.
    B. Encourage the client to do as little as possible.
    C. Meet basic needs if the client is confined to bed; prevent complications of bed rest.
    D. Assist with bladder or bowel training programs.
    E. Assist with range-of-motion exercises.
    F. Provide emotional support and encouragement.
    G. Report any changes in the person's mood or behaviour.

51. Infants and children may suffer brain damage from acquired brain injuries caused by:
    A. Conditions during birth
    B. Being shaken
    C. Childhood diseases
    D. Accidents

52. How can you help the client with pneumonia to breathe more easily and be more comfortable?
    A. Limit fluid intake.
    B. Position the client in high-Fowler's or semi-Fowler's position.
    C. Assist with oxygen therapy, as needed.

53. What damage can hypertension do to body organs?
    A. The heart may enlarge.
    B. Blood vessels in the brain may burst and cause a stroke.
    C. Blood vessels in the eyes may be damaged.
    D. Blood vessels in the kidneys (and other organs) may be damaged.

Copyright © 2018 Elsevier Canada, a division of Reed Elsevier Canada, Ltd.

54. Which risk factors of coronary artery disease can be changed by the client through lifestyle changes?
    A. Lack of exercise
    B. Excessive weight
    C. Smoking
    D. Excessive alcohol
    E. Stress
    F. Genetic link

55. What signs and symptoms would tell you a client is experiencing angina pectoris?
    A. Pain on the right side that may travel (radiate) to the jaw, neck, shoulders, back, and arms
    B. Shortness of breath
    C. Nausea
    D. Dry skin
    E. Dizziness or light-headedness
    F. Fatigue
    G. Palpitations

56. If a client is having a myocardial infarction, the signs and symptoms may include:
    A. Sudden, severe chest pain, usually on the right side
    B. Pain described as crushing, stabbing, or squeezing
    C. Pain that radiates to the neck and jaw, and down the arm or to the sides
    D. Pain that is more severe and lasts longer than angina
    E. Pain that is relieved by rest and nitroglycerin
    F. Indigestion
    G. Shortness of breath
    H. Nausea or vomiting
    I. Dizziness
    J. Perspiration
    K. Cyanosis
    L. Cold and clammy skin
    M. Low blood pressure
    N. Weak and irregular pulse

57. How is pain from angina relieved or avoided?
    A. Elective bypass surgery
    B. Resting when the pain begins
    C. Avoiding stress
    D. Avoiding other triggers (extreme cold or heat, heavy meals, alcohol, smoking)
    E. Taking nitroglycerin
    F. Reducing physical exertion

58. When you are caring for a client with acute renal failure, the care plan is likely to include which of the following instructions?
    A. Strain the urine every six hours
    B. Measure and record intake and urinary catheter output every hour
    C. Increase fluid intake
    D. Weigh the client daily using a different scale
    E. Provide frequent oral hygiene
    F. Meet basic needs if the client is confined to bed; prevent complications of bed rest
    G. Prevent infections

59. What are the signs and symptoms of hepatitis?
    A. Nausea, vomiting, and abdominal pain
    B. Light-coloured urine
    C. Jaundice
    D. Dark-coloured stools
    E. Muscle pain
    F. Increased energy
    G. Irritability
    H. Itching
    I. Diarrhea
    J. General aching in the joints, accompanied by redness and swelling

60. Some complications of diabetes mellitus include:
    A. Blindness
    B. Kidney disease
    C. Nerve damage
    D. Sexual dysfunction
    E. Circulatory disorders
    F. Stroke and heart attack
    G. Improved wound healing

Copyright © 2018 Elsevier Canada, a division of Reed Elsevier Canada, Ltd.

61. AIDS is spread by:
    A. Protected intercourse with an HIV-infected person
    B. Needle-sharing among IV drug users
    C. HIV-infected mothers to their babies at birth or during breastfeeding
    D. Infected body fluids (not including saliva, tears, urine, or sweat) coming into direct contact with broken skin
    E. Needle stick injuries
    F. Casual contact such as hugging

62. What signs and symptoms may occur with both hypoglycemia and hyperglycemia?
    A. Hunger
    B. Vision changes
    C. Headache
    D. Slow pulse
    E. High blood pressure
    F. Confusion
    G. Convulsions
    H. Loss of consciousness

MULTIPLE CHOICE

Circle the correct answer.

63. What is a helpful suggestion that you can give to a client who has pain associated with rheumatoid arthritis?
    A. Refrain from doing range-of-motion exercises.
    B. Refrain from drinking citrus juices.
    C. Follow your physician's recommendations in regard to heat and cold applications.
    D. Encourage the client to follow a diabetic diet.

64. Which of the following is a cause of osteoporosis?
    A. Excessive number of leukocytes in the blood.
    B. Lack of dietary calcium
    C. Lack of testosterone production
    D. Running marathon races

65. When caring for a client who had a recent hip replacement, which of these activities can cause the hip joint to dislocate?
    A. Abducting the affected leg
    B. Using an abductor splint or pillow between the legs when in bed
    C. Any activity that bends the hip joint by more than 90 degrees.
    D. Using a shower chair for bathing

66. Gangrene can occur because of:
    A. Joint immobility and inflammation
    B. Infection, injuries, and decreased circulation
    C. Poor body alignment and positioning
    D. Porous, brittle bones

67. A transient ischemic attack (TIA):
    A. Is another name for a stroke
    B. Occurs when blood supply to the brain is disrupted for a short period
    C. Occurs when blood pressure is elevated
    D. Occurs when there is high sugar in the blood

68. When caring for a client with a spinal cord injury, you would:
    A. Encourage the use of heating pads on the client's paralyzed limbs
    B. Follow bowel and bladder training programs with the client
    C. Limit the client's visitors
    D. Recommend a puréed diet for the client

69. You are caring for a client who has angina, and you find a bottle of tablets marked "Nitroglycerine" at the bedside. You should:
    A. Place them in a locked cabinet
    B. Tell the nurse
    C. Give them to the family to take home
    D. Make sure they remain where the client put them

Copyright © 2018 Elsevier Canada, a division of Reed Elsevier Canada, Ltd.

70. Which of these measures would be included in the treatment of a client with congestive heart failure?
    A. Measuring the client's weight daily before breakfast.
    B. Ensuring the client eats a diet high in salt
    C. Encouraging the client to exercise vigorously
    D. Encouraging the client to maintain a low-Fowler's position

71. Childhood communicable diseases are most commonly transmitted by:
    A. Airborne spread of or direct contact with respiratory secretions
    B. Direct contact with feces
    C. Direct contact with skin lesions
    D. Contact with a carrier

72. Which disease do the following signs and symptoms describe?
    Unusual mass or swelling, unexplained paleness or loss of energy, sudden tendency to bruise, persistent localized pain, or frequent headaches, especially with vomiting
    A. Stroke
    B. Emphysema
    C. Cancer
    D. Parkinson's disease

73. Which disease do the following signs and symptoms describe?
    Blurred or double vision, numbness and tingling, muscle weakness, difficulty speaking, dizziness, poor coordination, bladder problems
    A. Stroke
    B. Parkinson's disease
    C. Multiple sclerosis
    D. Emphysema

74. Which disease do the following signs and symptoms describe?
    Sudden weakness or numbness on one side of the body, impaired vision or loss of vision, loss of speech or trouble talking, loss of control of facial muscles, unexplained dizziness
    A. Stroke
    B. Parkinson's disease
    C. Multiple sclerosis
    D. Emphysema

75. Which disease do the following signs and symptoms describe?
    Enlarged alveoli, loss of elasticity in the walls of the alveoli, air remaining trapped in the alveoli during expiration, shortness of breath and "smoker's cough," barrel chest
    A. Stroke
    B. Parkinson's disease
    C. Multiple sclerosis
    D. Emphysema

76. Which disease do the following signs and symptoms describe?
    Mask-like facial expression, tremors, pill-rolling movements of the fingers, shuffling gait, impaired balance, stooped posture, stiff muscles, slurred or monotone speech, drooling
    A. Cancer
    B. Parkinson's disease
    C. Multiple sclerosis
    D. Emphysema

77. Which area of the body would be paralyzed if the client had a cervical spine injury?
    A. From the neck down
    B. One side of the body
    C. From the chest down
    D. From the waist down

78. Spinal cord injuries at the thoracic level (chest area) or lower may cause:
    A. Quadriplegia
    B. Paralysis on one side of the body
    C. Paraplegia
    D. Paralysis of one limb

Copyright © 2018 Elsevier Canada, a division of Reed Elsevier Canada, Ltd.

MATCHING

Match the disease process to the symptom or physical effect listed below:

A. *Chronic bronchitis*
B. *Emphysema*

79. _____ Person develops barrel chest

80. _____ Mucus and inflamed breathing passages obstruct airflow

81. _____ Walls of alveoli are less elastic

Match the correct term to the symptom or physical effect listed below:

A. *Hypoglycemia*
B. *Hyperglycemia*

82. _____ Trembling

83. _____ Nausea and vomiting

84. _____ Cold, clammy skin

85. _____ Flushed face

86. _____ Tiredness and fatigue

87. _____ Dizziness

88. _____ Dry skin

89. _____ Sweating

90. _____ Slow, laboured breathing

Match the type of diabetes mellitus with the age or situation when each type usually occurs.

91. _____ Type 1 diabetes

92. _____ Type 2 diabetes

93. _____ Gestational diabetes

A. Develops during pregnancy

B. Occurs most often in children and young adults

C. Usually develops in adulthood

Copyright © 2018 Elsevier Canada, a division of Reed Elsevier Canada, Ltd.

FILL IN THE BLANKS

94. Why does a client with osteoarthritis have more pain when standing and walking?

    _____ .

95. What type of arthritis occurs in children?

    _____

96. What are the goals in treating rheumatoid arthritis?
    a. _____
    b. _____
    c. _____

97. For each of these signs and symptoms that should be reported immediately if they occur to a client with a cast, explain the possible cause.
    a. Pain

       _____

    b. Swelling/tight cast

       _____

    c. Pale skin

       _____

    d. Cyanosis

       _____

    e. Odour

       _____

    f. Inability to move toes or fingers

       _____

    g. Numbness

       _____

    h. Temperature changes

       _____

    i. Drainage on or under cast

       _____

    j. Chills, fever, nausea, vomiting

       _____

98. When an extremity must be amputated because of gangrene, what areas of the client's life may be affected?
    a. _____
    b. _____
    c. _____

99. Why are older clients at higher risk for serious problems after a hip fracture?
    a. _____
    b. _____

Copyright © 2018 Elsevier Canada, a division of Reed Elsevier Canada, Ltd.

100. A client with Parkinson's disease may need assistance with:

a. _____

b. _____

c. _____

d. _____

101. A client with chronic obstructive pulmonary disease (COPD) must stop

_____.

102. How can you help a client with pneumonia to breathe more easily and be more comfortable?

a. _____

b. _____

c. _____

103. How are tuberculosis bacteria spread?

_____

104. What precautions to prevent infection should be used when caring for a client with tuberculosis?

a. _____

b. _____

105. When caring for a client with tuberculosis, how should you dispose of tissues?

a. In the home

_____

b. In a health care facility

_____

106. How do these risk factors affect hypertension?

a. Age

_____

b. Ethnicity

_____

c. Family history

_____

d. Obesity

_____

e. Stress

_____

f. Smoking

_____

g. Alcohol

_____

107. What measures could you use when caring for a client with heart failure?

a. _____

b. _____

c. _____

d. _____

e. _____

Copyright © 2018 Elsevier Canada, a division of Reed Elsevier Canada, Ltd.

108. Why are older clients with heart failure at risk for skin breakdown?
_____

109. If you are caring for a client who has renal calculi, you should encourage the client to drink about _____ per day.

110. With acute renal failure, recovery may take _____.

111. With chronic renal failure, the nephrons of the kidneys are _____.

112. Dialysis is done with chronic renal failure to remove _____.

113. What measures are used to care for a client in chronic renal failure?
   a. _____
   b. _____
   c. _____
   d. _____
   e. _____
   f. _____
   g. _____

114. Why is good foot care very important for a person with diabetes?
_____
_____
_____

115. To protect yourself from contracting hepatitis, you use _____.

116. Signs and symptoms of AIDS related to the following include:
   a. Skin _____
   _____
   b. Mouth and neck _____
   _____
   c. Mental status _____
   _____
   d. Digestive system _____
   _____

117. Why does a client with AIDS often develop other diseases?
_____

118. STDs may enter the body through many body areas such as the _____

Copyright © 2018 Elsevier Canada, a division of Reed Elsevier Canada, Ltd.

LABELLING

119. Colour the area that would be paralyzed if the person had a cervical spine injury.

120. Colour the area that would be paralyzed if the person had a lumbar spine injury.

Copyright © 2018 Elsevier Canada, a division of Reed Elsevier Canada, Ltd.

Developmental Disabilities and Disorders

TRUE OR FALSE

Circle T for true, or circle F for false.

1. T F People with a mild intellectual disability are slow to learn in school.

2. T F People with developmental disabilities do not have sexual urges.

3. T F All people with a developmental disability have the same amount of impairment.

4. T F Down syndrome causes some degree of intellectual disability in all affected people.

5. T F Cerebral palsy results from brain damage that occurs during birth.

6. T F Spastic cerebral palsy affects posture, balance, and movement.

7. T F Autism begins in early childhood.

8. T F Autism can be cured with appropriate therapies.

9. T F Children with myelomeningocele may learn to walk using braces or crutches.

10. T F If a child has hydrocephalus, intellectual disabilities and neurological damage will occur without treatment.

11. T F If a mother develops rubella (German measles) during pregnancy, the baby may have an intellectual disability.

12. T F Shaking a baby can cause intellectual disability.

Copyright © 2018 Elsevier Canada, a division of Reed Elsevier Canada, Ltd.

MULTIPLE RESPONSE

From the list below, choose all the correct answers.

13. What are some kinds of developmental disabilities?
    A. Intellectual disabilities
    B. Down syndrome
    C. Autism
    D. Cerebral palsy
    E. Chronic fatigue syndrome
    F. Spina bifida
    G. Fetal alcohol syndrome

14. What are some of the causes of intellectual disability?
    A. Abnormal genes inherited from one or both parents
    B. Missing or extra chromosomes
    C. Illness of mother during pregnancy
    D. Premature birth
    E. Alcohol or drug use during pregnancy
    F. Adequate nutrition
    G. Acquired brain injury

15. The Canadian Association for Community Living believes the following:
    A. Children with an intellectual disability should live with families and be integrated into regular schools whenever possible.
    B. Children with an intellectual disability should learn and play with others who do not have disabilities.
    C. Adults with an intellectual disability should control their own lives to the fullest extent possible.
    D. Adults with an intellectual disability should live in a long-term care facility or have choices and decisions about their care made by others.
    E. People with an intellectual disability have the right to privacy and to love and be loved.
    F. People with an intellectual disability should learn about sex, sexual abuse, and sexuality issues.

16. What are the physical characteristics of Down syndrome?
    A. Large head
    B. Oval-shaped eyes that slant upward
    C. Flat face
    D. Short, wide neck
    E. Small tongue
    F. Wide, flat nose
    G. Large ears
    H. Short stature
    I. Short, wide hands with stubby fingers
    J. Good muscle tone

17. What therapies will probably be needed for children and adults with Down syndrome?
    A. Speech therapy
    B. Language therapy
    C. Physiotherapy
    D. Occupational therapy

18. Infants at risk for cerebral palsy include those who:
    A. Have a high birth weight
    B. Do not cry in the first 5 minutes after birth
    C. Need mechanical ventilation
    D. Have bleeding in the brain
    E. Have heart, kidney, or spinal cord abnormalities
    F. Have blood problems
    G. Have seizures

19. What impairments may occur with cerebral palsy?
    A. Intellectual disability
    B. Learning disability
    C. Hearing impairments
    D. Speech impairments
    E. Vision impairments
    F. Bowel and bladder control problems
    G. Seizures
    H. Attention-deficit hyperactivity disorder
    I. Breathing problems

Copyright © 2018 Elsevier Canada, a division of Reed Elsevier Canada, Ltd.

20. Symptoms of attention-deficit hyperactivity disorder (ADHD) can include:
    A.   Becoming easily flustered and tense
    B.   A tendency toward addictive behaviours
    C.   Difficulty structuring time and setting priorities
    D.   Breath-holding and pouting behaviour
    E.   Difficulty completing tasks

21. What behaviours would you expect to see in a client with autism spectrum disorder (ASD)?
    A.   Poor speaking skills
    B.   Repeating words or phrases
    C.   Starting or maintaining conversation
    D.   Repeating body movements
    E.   Spending time with others
    F.   Showing little reaction to pain
    G.   Overreacting to noise and touch
    H.   Liking cuddling
    I.   Having frequent tantrums for no apparent reason
    J.   Forming strong attachment to a single item, idea, activity, or person
    K.   Needing routines
    L.   Fearing danger
    M.   Responding to others
    N.   Displaying aggressive or violent behaviour

22. What therapies are used to help the client with autism spectrum disorder (ASD)?
    A.   Behaviour modification
    B.   Speech and language therapy
    C.   Music, auditory, recreation, and sensory therapies
    D.   Occupational therapy
    E.   Surgical modification
    F.   Medication therapy
    G.   Diet therapy

MULTIPLE CHOICE

Circle the correct answer.

23. A client with epilepsy:
    A.   Can never drive a car
    B.   May be able to function normally with medication
    C.   Can never get a job
    D.   Is intellectually disabled

24. Hydrocephalus is treated by:
    A.   Medication
    B.   Closing the sac or pouch
    C.   Placing a shunt in the brain
    D.   Physiotherapy and occupational therapy

25. Certain body movements and body parts are affected by cerebral palsy (CP). Identify the correct term used to describe the loss of ability to move corresponding parts on both sides of the body.
    A.   Diplegia
    B.   Monoplegia
    C.   Hemiplegia
    D.   Quadriplegia

26. A client with cerebral palsy may have:
    A.   A large tongue
    B.   Short, wide hands
    C.   Involuntary movements
    D.   A small head

27. A client with autism spectrum disorder (ASD) may:
    A.   Show little reaction to pain
    B.   Have speech impairments
    C.   Have seizures
    D.   Drool

Copyright © 2018 Elsevier Canada, a division of Reed Elsevier Canada, Ltd.

MATCHING

Match the types of spina bifida with the correct description.

28. _____Part of the spinal column is contained in a sac

29. _____Spinal cord and nerves are usually normal; corrected with surgery

30. _____Defect in vertebrae closure but cannot be seen on outside of body

31. _____Pouch contains nerves and spinal cord; loss of function

A. Spina bifida occulta

B. Spina bifida cystica

C. Meningocele

D. Myelomeningocele

Match the three types of cerebral palsy to the correct description of muscle movements.

32. _____Spastic

33. _____Athetoid

34. _____Ataxic

A. Muscle tone is weak, and coordinating movement is difficult.

B. Movement is stiff and jerky, affecting one or both sides of the body.

C. Movement is involuntary and involves constant, slow weaving or withering motions in the trunk, arms, hands, legs, and feet.

FILL IN THE BLANKS

35. What physical disorders or problems often affect children with Down syndrome?

    a. _____

    b. _____

    c. At risk for _____

36. Lack of oxygen in early childhood can also cause cerebral palsy. The lack of oxygen can occur from

    a. _____

    b. _____

    c. _____

    d. _____

37. What activities of daily living are affected because of spastic movements with cerebral palsy?

    _____

Copyright © 2018 Elsevier Canada, a division of Reed Elsevier Canada, Ltd.

38. What functions are impaired with autism spectrum disorder?

    a. _____

    b. _____

    c. _____

39. What kind of impairment can occur with these disorders?
    a. Spina bifida occulta

    _____

    b. Meningocele

    _____

    c. Myelomeningocele

    _____

40. If the pressure inside the head of a child with hydrocephalus is not treated, what kinds of problems can result?

    a. _____

    b. _____

    c. _____

Copyright © 2018 Elsevier Canada, a division of Reed Elsevier Canada, Ltd.

CHAPTER 39

Speech and Language Disorders

TRUE OR FALSE

Circle T for true, or circle F for false.

1. **T** **F** Most older adults have apraxia.

2. **T** **F** Some people with aphasia cannot understand the message.

3. **T** **F** People with expressive aphasia are not aware of their mistakes when speaking.

4. **T** **F** Dysarthria is caused by weakness in the muscles used for speech.

5. **T** **F** Relationships between family members are not affected when someone has a speech disorder.

6. **T** **F** Shopping and cooking are not affected when someone has a communication problem.

7. **T** **F** Because you do not need to spend time on communication, you can take less time giving care to someone who cannot speak.

8. **T** **F** It is a help to the client to finish words for him.

9. **T** **F** Use positive statements rather than negative statements.

10. **T** **F** Aphasia is seldom permanent.

MULTIPLE RESPONSE

From the list below, choose all of the correct answers.

11. What can cause speech and language challenges?
    A. Genetic problems or conditions present at birth
    B. Poor eating habits
    C. Brain injury, which may be caused by accident, infection, drug abuse, stroke, and so on
    D. Disease
    E. Hearing loss
    F. Brain tumours
    G. Stress incontinence
    H. Problems involving the structures used for speech

Copyright © 2018 Elsevier Canada, a division of Reed Elsevier Canada, Ltd.

12. The basic types of aphasia (and their meanings) include:
    A. Receptive aphasia: difficulty speaking or writing
    B. Receptive aphasia: difficulty understanding written or spoken words
    C. Expressive aphasia: difficulty speaking or writing
    D. Motor aphasia: difficulty moving limbs
    E. Expressive–receptive aphasia (also known as global aphasia): difficulty speaking and understanding language

13. Which points describe *dysarthria*?
    A. Clients have difficulty speaking clearly because of weakness or paralysis in the muscles used to speak.
    B. Clients usually have slurred, slow, and soft speech.
    C. Clients often have problems forming words, spacing their words, and breathing while speaking.
    D. Clients cannot move the muscles used to speak.

14. What are some of the emotions people with speech and language disorders may experience?
    A. Frustration
    B. Depression
    C. Anger
    D. Low self-esteem
    E. Excitement
    F. Shame
    G. Guilt

15. How do you provide compassionate care to clients who have speech or language disorders?
    A. Address questions and comments to the client, not to others who are present.
    B. Do not force a client to talk in front of others.
    C. Never show impatience, frustration, or worry when a client is having problems speaking or understanding.
    D. Discourage communication. It will only make the client upset and frustrated.
    E. Limit the number of choices to help the client express preferences.

16. How can support workers show their respect for clients with speech or language disorders?
    A. By being encouraging and supportive
    B. By keeping private information confidential
    C. By learning to be comfortable with silence
    D. By taking extra time to explain procedures and not explaining all the steps at once
    E. By speaking slowly and clearly
    F. By being alert to signs the client has not understood you

Copyright © 2018 Elsevier Canada, a division of Reed Elsevier Canada, Ltd.

17. Some guidelines to effective communication with clients with speech or language disorders are:
    A. Minimize distractions by keeping the client alone as much as possible.
    B. Adjust the lighting; make sure the client can see your face clearly and that you can see the client's.
    C. Give the client your full attention; sit next to the client and speak into his ear.
    D. Ask the client questions to which you know the answer; this helps you become familiar with the client's speech.
    E. Determine the subject being discussed; look for nonverbal clues.
    F. Follow the client's lead; change your communication method as needed.
    G. Speak slowly, clearly, and in a normal tone of voice.
    H. Give the client time to respond; do not answer your own questions.
    I. Use simple words and short sentences; focus mainly on action words and words for people, places, and things.
    J. Be patient; repeat yourself as needed.
    K. Use positive statements.
    L. Use appropriate questioning and paraphrasing techniques; ask questions that require only a short answer or shake of the head, and summarize in your own words what the client has said.
    M. Try to speak without the use of gestures or pointing.
    N. Try other communication methods; follow the care plan and use writing and communication boards as needed.

MULTIPLE CHOICE

Circle the correct answer.

18. Mrs. Ekove can understand others but cannot speak. Which type of aphasia is she likely to have?
    A. Expressive aphasia
    B. Receptive aphasia
    C. Expressive–receptive aphasia
    D. Hemiplegia

19. After asking Mrs. Ekove a question, the support worker should:
    A. Allow time for her to process the question
    B. Expect an answer in a short time
    C. Repeat the question again immediately
    D. Ask if she is going to answer the question

20. To ensure that Mr. Ross understands what you have said, you should:
    A. Always have a witness when you speak to him
    B. Ask questions to see if he understood you
    C. Ask him to take notes while you speak
    D. Not bother to speak; instead, write things down and give him the note

21. Mrs. Faubert cannot speak. To communicate with her, you should:
    A. Use body language
    B. Shout slowly and distinctly
    C. Use sign language
    D. Follow the care plan

22. Which of the following is true in regard to electronic communication?
    A. These devices are not useful for assisting older adults to communicate.
    B. They are not recommended for clients with verbal-expression communication disorders.
    C. A male or female voice can be generated from the electronic aid.
    D. These are helpful only for clients with good eyesight.

Copyright © 2018 Elsevier Canada, a division of Reed Elsevier Canada, Ltd.

FILL IN THE BLANKS

23. Apraxia of speech means _____.

    People with this disorder _____

    _____

    _____.

24. Dysarthria means _____.

    People with this disorder _____

    _____

    _____

    _____.

Copyright © 2018 Elsevier Canada, a division of Reed Elsevier Canada, Ltd.

Hearing and Vision Disorders

TRUE OR FALSE

Circle T for true, or circle F for false.

1. **T   F**   *Presbyopia* is an age-related change that takes place in the eye.

2. **T   F**   Clients with a hearing impairment understand what you are saying if you exaggerate your words.

3. **T   F**   *Age-related macular degeneration* is damage to blood vessels in the retina as a result of diabetes.

4. **T   F**   Severe vision loss affects a client's physical, social, intellectual, and spiritual health.

5. **T   F**   Dogs can be specially trained to work with clients who have hearing loss.

6. **T   F**   Clients with hearing problems may avoid social situations because they cannot follow conversations.

7. **T   F**   Clients with hearing problems sometimes control conversations because they cannot hear if someone else has something to say.

8. **T   F**   Clients with hearing problems may get frustrated or irritable as they are under continual stress, trying to compensate for their hearing loss.

9. **T   F**   If you see a client with a guide dog or a white cane with a red tip, you should recognize that the client is blind.

MULTIPLE RESPONSE

From the list below, choose all of the correct answers.

10. Which of the following guidelines will help you to communicate better with a client with a hearing loss?
    A. Alert the client to your presence.
    B. Adjust the lighting so the client can see your face for lip reading.
    C. Increase background noise.
    D. Focus your attention on the client; if the client hears from only one ear, stand or sit on the side of the unaffected ear, and do not do other tasks while speaking to the client.
    E. Speak in a loud voice; do not shout, and do not cover your mouth when talking.
    F. Check communication aids; make sure the client is wearing hearing aids and eyeglasses, if used.
    G. Adjust your language; state the topic of conversation clearly, and use simple words and short sentences; say things in a different way if the client does not understand you.
    H. Use other communication methods (e.g., use body language or write key words on paper).
    I. Watch for signs of fatigue; avoid tiring the client.

11. What should you do if a hearing aid does not seem to work properly?
    A. Check if the hearing aid is on
    B. Check the battery position
    C. Insert a new battery if needed
    D. Clean the hearing aid with hot soapy water

12. Which are the correct steps to clean an artificial eye?
    A. Wash the eye with mild soap and warm water. Rinse well.
    B. Line a container with a tissue or with toilet paper.
    C. Fill the container with any cleaning solution.
    D. Label the container with the client's name and room number (if in a facility).
    E. Place the container in the drawer in the bedside stand or in another safe place as directed by the client.
    F. Wash the eye socket with hot soapy water. Use a washcloth or gauze square.
    G. Wash the eyelid with mild soap and warm water. Clean from the outer to the inner part of the eye.

13. Which of the following will assist you to care for a client with vision loss?
    A. Adjust the lighting to avoid glare; stand or sit in good light.
    B. Alert the client to your presence; identify yourself when you enter the room, and tell the person when you are leaving the room.
    C. Focus your attention on the client; do not turn or walk away while talking, and do not do other tasks while talking.
    D. Speak in a loud voice; speak slowly and clearly.
    E. Assist with walking.
    F. Assist with eating.
    G. Keep walkways clear and free of clutter.
    H. Keep doors partially opened.

14. Which of these is a responsibility of a support worker?
    A. Checking the battery position in a hearing aid
    B. Cleaning eyeglasses with warm water
    C. Assisting a client to remove an artificial eye
    D. Removing wax from a client's ear canal

Copyright © 2018 Elsevier Canada, a division of Reed Elsevier Canada, Ltd.

MULTIPLE CHOICE

Circle the correct answers.

15. Which disorder may cause vertigo?
    A.   Glaucoma
    B.   Otitis media
    C.   Ménière's disease
    D.   Cataracts

16. Which of these actions by a client indicate that the client has a hearing loss?
    A.   Speaking very softly
    B.   Asking for words to be repeated
    C.   Pronouncing words very clearly
    D.   Answering questions appropriately while watching television

17. What is the most common cause of blindness in clients over 50?
    A.   Cataracts
    B.   Age-related macular degeneration
    C.   Vertigo
    D.   Otitis media

18. Symptoms of retinal detachment include:
    A.   Yellow liquid discharge from the affected eye
    B.   A reported loss of central vision
    C.   Reports of seeing yellow halos around people
    D.   Flashing lights in the corner of the affected eye

19. When a client is legally blind, she:
    A.   Cannot sense light and has no usable vision
    B.   Can sense some light but has no usable vision
    C.   Has some usable vision but cannot read newsprint
    D.   Sees at 6 metres what a person with normal vision sees at 60 metres

20. What disease do the following statements describe?
    • *Pressure within the eye is increased.*
    • *It has a gradual or sudden onset.*
    • *The signs and symptoms include tunnel vision, blurred vision, and blue–green halos around lights.*
    • *With a sudden onset, there also is severe eye pain, nausea, and vomiting.*
    A.   Ménière's disease
    B.   Glaucoma
    C.   Cataract
    D.   Brain tumour

21. What disease do the following statements describe?
    • *Involves increased fluid in the inner ear.*
    • *Symptoms are vertigo, tinnitus, and hearing loss.*
    A.   Ménière's disease
    B.   Glaucoma
    C.   Cataract
    D.   Brain tumour

22. What disorder do the following statements describe?
    • *The lens becomes opaque.*
    • *A gradual blurring and dimming of vision occurs.*
    • *It can occur in one or both eyes.*
    • *Aging is the most common cause.*
    A.   Ménière's disease
    B.   Glaucoma
    C.   Cataract
    D.   Brain tumour

Copyright © 2018 Elsevier Canada, a division of Reed Elsevier Canada, Ltd.

MATCHING

Match the term related to hearing and vision problems with the correct definition.

23. _____Dizziness

24. _____Ringing in the ears

25. _____Method of writing using raised dots

26. _____Infection of the middle ear

A. Otitis media

B. Tinnitus

C. Vertigo

D. Braille

FILL IN THE BLANKS

27. Explain why the following behaviours may occur in clients with hearing problems.
    a. Avoids social situations

    _____

    b. Controls conversations

    _____

    c. Fatigue, frustration, irritability

    _____

28. What should you do to clean and store eyeglasses?
    a. Cleaning

    _____

    b. Storage

    _____

29. If you see a client with a guide dog or a white cane with a red tip, you should recognize that the client is _____.

Copyright © 2018 Elsevier Canada, a division of Reed Elsevier Canada, Ltd.

Oxygen Needs

TRUE OR FALSE

Circle T for true, or circle F for false.

1. T   F   The sensor for the pulse oximeter is used only on the fingers.

2. T   F   The doctor must order oxygen because oxygen is considered a drug.

3. T   F   The support worker is responsible for setting up a client's oxygen.

4. T   F   The type of device used to deliver oxygen is decided by the nurse.

5. T   F   A thoracentesis is a procedure in which lung tissue is removed.

6. T   F   A pulmonary function test measures the amount of oxygen in the client's blood.

7. T   F   Frequent oral hygiene should be given when the client is receiving oxygen therapy.

8. T   F   Tracheostomy tubes usually consist of three parts.

9. T   F   A cover is placed over the tracheostomy opening when the client is outside to prevent dust, insects, and other small particles from entering the stoma.

10. T   F   Suctioning the upper airway may be done through the mouth and pharynx or the nose and pharynx.

11. T   F   Suctioning should only be performed daily.

12. T   F   A clean (not sterile) catheter is used for oro-pharyngeal suctioning.

13. T   F   Support workers may change the settings on a mechanical ventilator as needed.

14. T   F   When a client has chest tubes, the drainage system is kept above the level of the client's chest.

15. T   F   Petrolatum gauze is kept at the bedside to cover the insertion site if a chest tube comes out.

Copyright © 2018 Elsevier Canada, a division of Reed Elsevier Canada, Ltd.

16. **T   F**   In the blood, hemoglobin contained within the red blood cells picks up oxygen in the lungs and carries it to the cells.

17. **T   F**   If the client is wearing dark nail polish, you should remove it when you want to use the pulse oximeter.

18. **T   F**   Gloves are worn to prevent the spread of infection when collecting a sputum specimen because sputum is a bodily fluid.

19. **T   F**   If you observe that the oxygen rate is not set at the rate the nurse stated, you need to adjust it immediately.

20. **T   F**   Signs of irritation are evident on the client's arms when he or she is wearing an oxygen cannula or mask.

21. **T   F**   A humidifier is often used in oxygen administration to humidify the oxygen so it will not dry the mucous membranes in the client's airway.

22. **T   F**   Coughing and deep-breathing exercises help to prevent hyperventilation.

MULTIPLE RESPONSE

From the list below, choose all of the correct answers.

23. What processes are involved in the function of the respiratory system?
    A. Air moves into and out of the lungs.
    B. Carbon dioxide is absorbed into the bloodstream from the lungs.
    C. Oxygen (O_2) and carbon dioxide (CO_2) are exchanged at the alveoli.
    D. The blood transports O_2 to the cells and removes CO_2 from them.

24. What signs and symptoms would tell you the client has hypoxia?
    A. Restlessness
    B. Constipation
    C. Dizziness
    D. Disorientation
    E. Confusion
    F. Behaviour and personality changes
    G. Increased ability to concentrate and follow directions
    H. Apprehension
    I. Anxiety
    J. Fatigue
    K. Agitation
    L. Decreased pulse rate
    M. Decreased rate and depth of respirations
    N. Often leaning forward when in a sitting position
    O. Cyanosis
    P. Dyspnea

25. When a pulse oximeter is used, what should be reported and recorded?
    A. If you think the machine is not working
    B. What the client was doing at the time of the measurement
    C. Oxygen flow rate and the device used
    D. Reason for the measurement (routine or change in the client's condition)
    E. Other observations

26. How is the client instructed to exhale during coughing and deep-breathing exercises?
    A. "Exhale slowly through pursed lips."
    B. "Exhale in short, forceful puffs."
    C. "Exhale until you feel light-headed."
    D. "Exhale until your ribs move as far down as possible."

27. What rules should you follow when handling the tubing for oxygen administration?
    A. Secure connecting tubing (i.e., nasal cannula) in place.
    B. Make sure there are no kinks in the tubing.
    C. Tape or pin the tubing to the client's garment according to employer policy.
    D. Make sure the client does not lie on any part of the tubing.
    E. Never handle the tubing without gloves.

Copyright © 2018 Elsevier Canada, a division of Reed Elsevier Canada, Ltd.

28. What fire safety rules should be followed if oxygen is in use?
    A. Place "No Smoking" signs in the room and on the room door.
    B. Remove materials from the room that ignite easily.
    C. Turn off electrical items before unplugging them.
    D. Use electrical equipment that is in good repair.
    E. Do not use materials that cause static electricity (wool and synthetic fabrics).
    F. Know the location of fire extinguishers and how to use them.
    G. If a fire occurs, turn off the oxygen. Then get the client to safety.
    H. Remind the client and family members about oxygen safety. Report safety hazards immediately.

29. How can you assist the nurse in caring for clients with artificial airways?
    A. By checking vital signs
    B. By observing the client for signs of hypoxia and other respiratory problems
    C. By reporting if an artificial airway comes out or is dislodged
    D. By providing oral hygiene twice a day

30. What are the parts of a tracheostomy tube?
    A. Outer cannula
    B. Middle cannula
    C. Inner cannula
    D. Obturator
    E. Respirator

31. When you are caring for a client with a tracheostomy, you should call the nurse if:
    A. The client shows signs and symptoms of hypoxia
    B. The client shows signs of respiratory distress
    C. The outer cannula comes out
    D. The client must urinate

32. What measures are implemented to prevent aspiration in a client with a tracheostomy?
    A. Make sure dressings do not have loose gauze or lint.
    B. Instruct the client to breathe through his nose.
    C. Make sure the stoma is not covered with plastic, leather, or similar materials.
    D. Instruct the client to take only showers.
    E. Make sure the client is helped with shampooing so that water does not enter the stoma.
    F. Instruct the client that swimming is not allowed.
    G. Make sure the client wears medical alert jewellery and carries a medical alert ID card.

33. What observations should you report to a nurse when assisting with suctioning a client?
    A. An increase in pulse rate
    B. Irregular cardiac rhythms
    C. A drop or rise in blood pressure
    D. Respiratory distress

34. When caring for a client with chest tubes, what information should be observed and reported to the nurse?
    A. Changes in vital signs
    B. Signs and symptoms of hypoxia and respiratory distress
    C. Complaints of pain or difficulty breathing
    D. A decrease in chest drainage
    E. Bubbling in the drainage system increasing, decreasing, or stopping
    F. Any part of the system being loose or disconnected
    G. A chest tube coming out

35. While caring for a client with chest tubes, one of the chest tubes falls out. After you call for help, what should you do next?
    A. Cover the insertion site with sterile petrolatum gauze
    B. Ask the client to hold his or her breath
    C. Keep the client in a supine position
    D. Stay with the client, and then follow the nurse's directions

MULTIPLE CHOICE

Circle the correct answer.

36. A pulse oximeter is used to measure:
    A. The oxygen concentration in arterial blood
    B. The pulse rate
    C. The oxygen concentration in the lungs
    D. The amount of oxygen in the blood

37. Which of these procedures may be done by a support worker?
    A. Administering oxygen therapy
    B. Suctioning
    C. Collecting a sputum specimen
    D. Performing tracheostomy care

38. When is the best time to collect a sputum specimen?
    A. At mealtime
    B. Early in the morning
    C. At bedtime
    D. After using mouthwash

39. What position is often preferred by clients with difficulty breathing?
    A. Lying on one side
    B. Supine position
    C. Orthopneic position
    D. Prone position

40. Which of these statements is true about administering oxygen with a face mask?
    A. The mask can irritate the throat.
    B. You need to listen carefully when the client who is wearing a mask is trying to speak. .
    C. The client may eat and drink while the mask is in place.
    D. Oral hygiene is not necessary when a client is receiving oxygen through a mask.

41. The acronym "SOBOE" stands for:
    A. Suction once by oxygen employee
    B. Sputum obtained by obturator extension
    C. Sudden oxygen bradypnea outpatient emergency
    D. Short of breath on exertion

42. When the nurse is giving tracheostomy care, the support worker may be asked to assist when the ties are removed by:
    A. Holding the inner cannula in place
    B. Cleaning the outer cannula
    C. Cleaning the stoma
    D. Suctioning the tracheostomy

43. Which of the following would be the responsibility of the support worker with a client on a mechanical ventilator?
    A. Resetting the alarm if it rings
    B. Performing suctioning whenever the breathing tube is plugged
    C. Carefully changing the oxygen tubing
    D. Using established hand or eye signals for "yes" and "no"

44. Mrs. Doronsulic's respiration rate is 34 breaths per minute. This is called:
    A. Eupnea
    B. Bradypnea
    C. Tachypnea
    D. Apnea

45. Which physical condition may *most likely* contribute to Mrs. Tleen's difficulty breathing?
    A. Diabetes
    B. Epilepsy
    C. Emphysema
    D. Glaucoma

46. Narcotic pain medication can affect breathing by causing:
    A. The respiration rate to increase
    B. Thickened mucus in the lungs
    C. Nasal congestion and sinus problems
    D. A suppressed respiration rate and breathing that is shallower than normal

Copyright © 2018 Elsevier Canada, a division of Reed Elsevier Canada, Ltd.

MATCHING

Match the name of each type of artificial airway with the correct description.

47. An artificial airway inserted through the mouth and into the pharynx

48. An artificial airway inserted through a nostril and into the pharynx

49. An artificial airway inserted through the mouth or nose and into the trachea

50. An artificial airway inserted through a surgical incision into the trachea

A. Tracheostomy tube

B. Endotracheal tube

C. Naso-pharyngeal airway

D. Oro-pharyngeal airway

Match each test with the correct description.

51. _____ Measures the amount of air moving in and out of the lungs

52. _____ Allows the doctor to inspect the trachea and bronchi

53. _____ Punctures and aspirates air or fluid from the pleura

54. _____ Evaluates changes in the lungs

55. _____ Radioactive gas is inhaled, allowing the physician to see what areas are not getting air or blood

56. _____ Laboratory test that measures the amount of oxygen in the blood

A. Chest X-ray

B. Lung scan

C. Bronchoscopy

D. Thoracentesis

E. Pulmonary function tests

F. Arterial blood gases

FILL IN THE BLANKS

57. Explain how these factors affect oxygen needs.
    a. Respiratory system

    _____

    b. Cardiovascular system

    _____

    c. Red blood cell count

    _____

    d. Nervous system

    _____

Copyright © 2018 Elsevier Canada, a division of Reed Elsevier Canada, Ltd.

e. Aging

_____

f. Exercise

_____

g. Fever

_____

h. Pain

_____

i. Drugs

_____

j. Smoking

_____

k. Allergies

_____

l. Pollutant exposure

_____

m. Nutrition

_____

n. Alcohol

_____

58. Coughing and deep-breathing exercises help to prevent _____ and

_____.

59. Describe each of these oxygen sources.

a. Wall outlet _____

b. Oxygen tank _____

c. Oxygen concentrator _____

60. Describe the following devices used to deliver oxygen.
a. Simple face mask

_____

b. Partial-rebreather mask

_____

Copyright © 2018 Elsevier Canada, a division of Reed Elsevier Canada, Ltd.

c. Non-rebreather mask

_____

d. Venturi mask

_____

61. What should you do if the oxygen humidifier is bubbling?

_____

62. Where should the support worker check for signs of irritation from the oxygen cannula or mask?

_____

63. How can the person with an artificial airway communicate with you?

_____

_____

64. When assisting with suctioning, the support worker may check the person's pulse, respirations, and pulse oximeter _____, _____, and _____ the procedure.

65. When the support worker is assisting with suctioning, the following should be reported to the nurse:

a. _____

b. _____

c. _____

d. _____

e. _____

66. An Ambu bag is used to _____ before _____ to prevent or treat hypoxia.

67. Why is it important to keep the call bell within reach and answer it promptly when you are caring for a person with mechanical ventilation?

_____

_____

Copyright © 2018 Elsevier Canada, a division of Reed Elsevier Canada, Ltd.

CROSSWORD

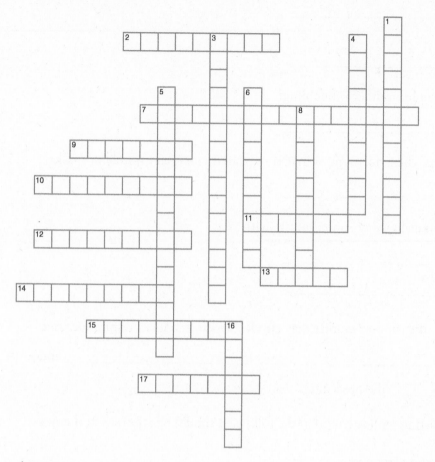

Across

2. Rapid breathing; respirations are usually more than 24 per minute

7. Respirations that are rapid and deeper than normal

9. Process of withdrawing or sucking up fluids (secretions)

10. Slow breathing; respirations are fewer than 12 per minute

11. Expectorated mucus

12. Below the normal level of oxygen in the blood

13. Lack or absence of breathing

14. Harmful chemical or substance in the air or water

15. Being able to breathe deeply and comfortably only while sitting or standing

17. Difficult, laboured, or painful breathing

Down

1. Collection of air in the pleural space

3. Escape and collection of fluid in the pleural space (2 words)

4. Collection of blood in the pleural space

5. Respirations that are slow, shallow, and sometimes irregular

6. Bloody sputum

8. Process of inserting an artificial airway

16. Sensitivity to a substance that causes the body to react with signs and symptoms

Copyright © 2018 Elsevier Canada, a division of Reed Elsevier Canada, Ltd.

Home Management

TRUE OR FALSE

Circle T for true, or circle F for false.

1. **T** **F** Work from dirtiest to cleanest.

2. **T** **F** Dust from higher surfaces to lower surfaces.

3. **T** **F** The use of gloves is not required when cleaning in a client's home.

4. **T** **F** It is safe to use any cleaner in the bathroom.

5. **T** **F** A client recovering from surgery may need extra cleaning done in the bathroom.

6. **T** **F** Baking soda will remove stains.

7. **T** **F** Any type of liquid soap can be used in the dishwasher.

8. **T** **F** Sort clothing by colour before washing.

9. **T** **F** Stained items should be soaked in bleach for 10 minutes before washing.

10. **T** **F** Some cleaners can scratch surfaces so read product labels carefully.

11. **T** **F** It is safe to mix chlorine bleach and ammonia to make a stronger cleaner.

MULTIPLE RESPONSE

From the list below, choose all of the correct answers.

12. To complete home management tasks, you need to use your time wisely. Identify the points below that will help you.
    A. Identify priorities.
    B. Establish a routine.
    C. Use your time well—start with tasks that have a waiting period or run automatically, and then go on to other tasks.
    D. Finish tasks, and put items away.
    E. Set time limits for each task.
    F. If one task takes too long, switch tasks. Watch the clock.
    G. Put the client's needs first.

13. To remove urine stains, you should:
    A. Rinse the stained item in hot water
    B. Soak the item in a solution of 1 L warm water, 2 mL liquid handwashing soap, and 15 mL bleach for 30 minutes
    C. Rinse the item in cool water
    D. Soak the item in a solution of 1 L warm water and 15 mL vinegar for 1 hour
    E. With permission, machine-wash the item with chlorine bleach and detergent. Dry as usual.

Copyright © 2018 Elsevier Canada, a division of Reed Elsevier Canada, Ltd.

14. Your goal when doing laundry is:
     A. To clean items
     B. Not to damage items
     C. To entertain the client

15. When cleaning kitchens, you should remember the following:
     A. Pour dirty or contaminated liquids down the kitchen sink only.
     B. Use one cloth for counters, another for wiping floors, and another for dishes.
     C. Use dishcloths to dry your hands.
     D. Change cloths daily as needed. Wash in bleach and hot water.
     E. Use paper towels for all tasks when possible.
     F. Clean outside the microwave after every use.
     G. Do not put soiled diapers into the kitchen garbage.

16. What can you do to decrease microbes in the bathroom?
     A. Remove and dispose of hair from the sink, tub, or shower.
     B. Flush the toilet with the seat down to prevent splashing.
     C. Rinse the sink after it has been used for washing, shaving, or oral hygiene.
     D. Hang damp towels and bath mats up to dry. Spread them out.
     E. Wash bath mats, the wastebasket, and the laundry hamper every week.
     F. Close shower doors.
     G. Let the bathtub or shower drip dry after use.
     H. Flush dirty or contaminated liquids down the toilet only.

17. Cleaning products can cause harm if not used properly. Remember to:
     A. Read all labels carefully
     B. Never mix cleaning products
     C. Wear latex gloves
     D. Never use products in unlabelled containers
     E. Store products in their original containers
     F. Keep cleaning products away from food
     G. Keep cleaning products out of reach of children and adults with dementia
     H. Use products only for their intended purpose
     I. Keep aerosol cans away from heat sources
     J. Ask the client before using a strong cleaner on a surface
     K. Rinse away strong, abrasive cleaners immediately after use
     L. Scrub vigorously when cleaning

18. What are some general cleaning guidelines?
     A. Clear away clutter.
     B. Work from lower to higher.
     C. Work from near to far.
     D. Work from dry to wet.
     E. Work from dirtiest to cleanest.
     F. Change cloths and water frequently.
     G. Use a dry cloth for dusting.
     H. Rinse and dry washed surfaces.
     I. Avoid soiling a clean area.

MULTIPLE CHOICE

Circle the correct answer.

19. When should spills and splashes be cleaned up?
     A. After meals
     B. Weekly
     C. Before you leave for the day
     D. Immediately

Copyright © 2018 Elsevier Canada, a division of Reed Elsevier Canada, Ltd.

20. Which statement about laundry care is true?
    A. All clothing should be ironed.
    B. All whites should be washed together.
    C. All whites are washed in hot water.
    D. Care label instructions should be followed.

21. You notice the client's clothing is missing care labels. What should you do?
    A. Ask the client for washing guidance.
    B. Guess how each article should be washed.
    C. Wash everything by hand.
    D. Wash everything in cold water.

MATCHING

Match each laundry symbol to its meaning.

24. Dry clean.

25. Handwash gently in cool water.

26. Machine-wash in hot water.

27. Use chlorine bleach with care.

28. Do not iron or press.

29. Hang to dry after removing excess water.

22. Why should cleaning products never be mixed together?
    A. Mixing chemicals reduces their cleaning effect.
    B. Cleaners may become toxic if mixed.
    C. Mixed chemicals can stain your hands.
    D. Mixing chemicals might make the article dirtier.

23. Which statement on food handling is true?
    A. Always wear gloves while cooking.
    B. Garbage should be disposed of weekly.
    C. Leftover food should be refrigerated immediately.
    D. Season the client's food to your taste.

A.

B.

C.

D.

E.

F.

Copyright © 2018 Elsevier Canada, a division of Reed Elsevier Canada, Ltd.

Assisting With Medications

TRUE OR FALSE

Circle T for true, or circle F for false.

1. **T   F**   An *elixir* is medication dissolved in a concentrated sugar solution.

2. **T   F**   It is your responsibility to ensure that your clients know about the side effects that can occur when they take their medications.

3. **T   F**   Part of your responsibility is to fill your client's pillbox each week.

4. **T   F**   To make a suppository more comfortable for insertion, apply petroleum jelly to it before handing it to the client.

5. **T   F**   A lozenge is a form of medication.

6. **T   F**   Some medications have to be taken on an empty stomach.

7. **T   F**   You must follow your agency's policies in regard to signing medication administration records (MARs).

8. **T   F**   Medication on transdermal discs is absorbed over 24 hours.

9. **T   F**   You may purchase over-the-counter medications for your client if requested to do so because these are not prescription drugs.

10. **T   F**   Dispensing medications is beyond your scope of practice.

MULTIPLE RESPONSE

From the list below, choose all of the correct answers.

11. Your role in assisting with medications may involve:
    A.   Reminding the client to take a medication
    B.   Bringing medication containers to the client
    C.   Bringing prepoured medications, pre-filled syringes, or pillboxes to the client
    D.   Reading the prescription label to the client
    E.   Loosening or removing container lids or opening blister packs
    F.   Checking the dosage against the medication label
    G.   Providing water or other fluids as needed
    H.   Phoning the client's family doctor for prescription refills
    I.   Supervising the client as she pours the medication into her hand, measuring spoon, or cup

12. A side effect of a medication:
    A. Is a response that occurs along with the main desired response to the medication
    B. May be predictable or unpredictable
    C. Is usually insignificant so you will not have to look for side effects

13. Which information is contained in most MARs?
    A. The client's name
    B. The client's medication allergies
    C. The name, dose, and administration instructions for each medication
    D. Why the client is taking the medication and what the side effects are
    E. A place to sign or initial after administering the medication

14. Medications should be stored:
    A. In a special place just for the person's medications
    B. In a warm place, such as in a cupboard over the stove
    C. Out of reach of children and adults with dementia
    D. In the original labelled container, with the lid tightly closed
    E. According to any special storage instructions

15. Some of the "rights" of assisting with medications include:
    A. The right reasons for taking the medication
    B. The right medication
    C. The right dose
    D. The right route
    E. The right time zone
    F. The right documentation
    G. The right expiration date
    H. The right doctor

16. Medication particles suspended in air or gas and inhaled through the lungs is called a:
    A. Puffer
    B. Suspension
    C. Inhaler
    D. Aerosol

17. If the medication is to dissolve under the client's tongue, you should:
    A. Place the medication under the tongue with your fingers
    B. Ask the client to close his or her mouth and let the medication dissolve
    C. Remind the client not to chew or swallow the medication
    D. Provide warm food or fluids to assist in dissolving the medication

18. What information is included on a prescription label?
    A. Pharmacy name
    B. Date filled
    C. Prescription warning labels
    D. Cost of the medication
    E. Physician's name
    F. Number of times the prescription can be refilled
    G. Drug name and dose
    H. Side effects of the medication
    I. Client's name
    J. Client's address

MULTIPLE CHOICE

Circle the correct answer.

19. Mrs. Smythe, one of your clients, is taking an antihistamine and drinking alcohol. What should you do first?
    A. Discuss the situation with your supervisor
    B. Throw away the rest of your client's alcohol
    C. Ask your client if she wants to die by suicide
    D. Observe the client for any more drinking

20. You have been assigned to apply Mrs. Smythe's prescription ointment for a rash on her back. What should you do first?
    A. Provide privacy for the client
    B. Put on a disposable glove
    C. Wash her skin well and dry it
    D. Check the MAR for all of the rights

Copyright © 2018 Elsevier Canada, a division of Reed Elsevier Canada, Ltd.

21. What is true about transdermal patches?
    A. They have medication that is absorbed through mucous membranes.
    B. They can leak easily, so they need to be covered up with a bandage.
    C. One must be removed before another one can be applied.
    D. They must be rubbed between your hands to activate the medication.

22. What is true about medication suspensions? They:
    A. Are always taken orally
    B. Need to be shaken well before being poured
    C. Usually are dissolved in alcohol
    D. Must be absorbed under the client's tongue

23. Your client cannot open the jar of her aspirin bottle and asks you to do it for her. Which is the most appropriate action to take?
    A. You open her bottle as requested and give it to her.
    B. Tell her that support workers are not allowed to do this.
    C. Check with your supervisor first if you are allowed.
    D. Check the client's medication administration records (MARs) as well as her care plan first.

24. A dosette is meant to:
    A. Remind clients when to take their medications
    B. Prevent the medication from going stale
    C. Protect the medication from exposure to heat
    D. Keep the medication clean and germ-free

25. A sublingual medication is:
    A. Digested in the client's small intestine
    B. Dissolved in the client's rectum
    C. Absorbed in the client's skin
    D. Dissolved under the client's tongue

26. A metered-dose inhaler is used for:
    A. Medications that are narcotics and under lock and key
    B. Children's medications
    C. Medications that must be inhaled into the lungs
    D. Drug addicts who might overdose easily

27. When working in home care, what should the support worker do with the MAR?
    A. Keep it in her car
    B. Keep it in the client's record at the client's home
    C. Keep it with the support worker's employer
    D. Discard it at the end of each day

Copyright © 2018 Elsevier Canada, a division of Reed Elsevier Canada, Ltd.

MATCHING

Match the abbreviation with the meaning.

28. _____ By mouth   A. bid

29. _____ Per rectum   B. hs

30. _____ Every hour   C. NPO

31. _____ Twice a day   D. PO

32. _____ Every 2 hours   E. qid

33. _____ Four times a day   F. pr

34. _____ Sublingual   G. qd

35. _____ Nothing by mouth   H. qh

36. _____ Hours of sleep   I. q2h

37. _____ Every day   J. sl

Match the medication route with its description.

38. _____ Taken by mouth and swallowed   A. Oral

39. _____ Applied to the skin or mucous membranes   B. Sublingual

40. _____ Breathed in through the mouth or nose   C. Parenteral

41. _____ Placed under the tongue and absorbed into the body   D. Inhalant

42. _____ Injected by a needle into a muscle, a vein, or under the skin   E. Topical

Copyright © 2018 Elsevier Canada, a division of Reed Elsevier Canada, Ltd.

FILL IN THE BLANKS

43. Medications come in many forms. List three and give an example of each.

a. _____

_____

b. _____

_____

c. _____

_____

Copyright © 2018 Elsevier Canada, a division of Reed Elsevier Canada, Ltd.

Heat and Cold Applications

TRUE OR FALSE

Circle T for true, or circle F for false.

1. **T** **F** Bags that contain beans or wheat should always be shaken thoroughly before being heated.

2. **T** **F** Applying cold to a body area will constrict blood flow to that area.

3. **T** **F** If the skin is pink, it would be described as being "cyanotic."

4. **T** **F** A *sitz* bath is a warm soak for sore hands and wrists.

5. **T** **F** Support workers can generally apply heat and cold packs to clients.

6. **T** **F** Moist heat usually penetrates more deeply than dry heat.

7. **T** **F** Applying a cold pack for too long can cause the underlying skin to burn.

8. **T** **F** Short-term heat applications affect blood vessels by making them constrict (or become narrow).

9. **T** **F** Heat or cold should be applied at 25-minute intervals.

10. **T** **F** You should check the skin every 15 minutes when moist heat or cold compresses are in place.

11. **T** **F** A *sitz* bath is a type of soak used to clean and soothe perineal or anal wounds.

12. **T** **F** Never apply a heat pack without covering the pack first.

MULTIPLE RESPONSE

From the list below, choose all of the correct answers.

13. How does dilation of the blood vessels to an area help in healing?
    A. More blood flows through the vessels and therefore tissues have more oxygen and nutrients for healing.
    B. The dilated blood vessels aid in digestion and make the client feel more relaxed.
    C. Excess fluid and wastes are removed from the area faster, helping to reduce pain and swelling and helping the muscles to relax.

Copyright © 2018 Elsevier Canada, a division of Reed Elsevier Canada, Ltd.

14. Heat applications are used to:
    A. Improve muscle tension
    B. Promote healing
    C. Relieve pain
    D. Reduce tissue swelling
    E. Increase joint stiffness
    F. Improve muscle strength and endurance

15. Which people or groups of people are at risk for burns from heat applications?
    A. People with metal implants
    B. Young children
    C. Older adults
    D. Dark-skinned people
    E. People who have decreased sensation (e.g., people with diabetes, spinal cord injuries, or stroke)
    F. People with dementia or confusion
    G. Infants

16. When working in home care, what can you use to apply ice?
    A. Ice bag
    B. Ice collar
    C. Ice cube tray
    D. Ice glove

17. What are the signs of complications when applying heat or cold?
    A. Complaints of discomfort, pain, numbness, or burning
    B. Excessive redness
    C. Blisters
    D. Pink skin
    E. Cyanosis
    F. Shivering

18. What guidelines should be followed for applying heat or cold?
    A. Apply only when ordered by a professional, allowed by your employer, and assigned to do so.
    B. Know how to use the equipment.
    C. Measure the temperature of moist applications after applying.
    D. Follow employer policies for safe temperature ranges.
    E. Do not apply hot applications above 49.1°C.
    F. Ask your supervisor what the temperature of the application should be.
    G. Know the precise site for the application.
    H. Before applying moist heat or cold applications, cover them with a flannel or terrycloth cover, towel, or pillowcase.
    I. Leave at-risk clients unattended only for short periods of time.
    J. Observe the skin for signs of complications. If any signs are observed, immediately remove the application and report to your supervisor.
    K. Observe for changes in the client's behaviour that may indicate sleepiness.
    L. Remind the client not to change the temperature of the application.
    M. Prevent chills. Cover the client with a blanket or robe. Control room drafts.
    N. Ask your supervisor how long to leave the application in place. Carefully watch the time.
    O. Applications are left on for no more than 25 minutes.
    P. Follow Standard Practices.

Copyright © 2018 Elsevier Canada, a division of Reed Elsevier Canada, Ltd.

MULTIPLE CHOICE

Circle the correct answer.

19. Which of these factors may make a client more susceptible to burns?
    A. Respiratory disorders
    B. Dehydration
    C. Circulatory disorders
    D. Infections

20. Heat should not be applied to which of these areas?
    A. Metal hip and knee replacements
    B. Joints
    C. Soft tissues
    D. Old fractures

21. A sitz bath may cause the client to feel weak or faint because:
    A. The bath increases pain in the area
    B. Blood flow increases in the pelvic area, and less blood flows to other body parts
    C. Blood flow decreases in the pelvic area, and more blood flows to other body parts
    D. The client becomes chilled

22. You applied a commercial cold pack to Jane's ankle as instructed in her care plan. After 3 minutes, she complains of extreme pain to the area. What should you do first?
    A. Check it after another 2 minutes.
    B. Notify your supervisor.
    C. Take her pulse in that area.
    D. Remove the cold pack.

23. Why are people with thin skin at increased risk for burns with heat and cold applications?
    A. They have better circulation than people with thicker skin.
    B. They lack enough of a protective adipose layer.
    C. They usually have taken better care of their skin.
    D. They lack feeling to their skin.

24. Heat and cold applications must be covered before being applied to a client's skin. Which is the best explanation for why this is done?
    A. It protects the heat and cold pack from wear and tear.
    B. It keeps the heat and cold pack cleaner and free of germs.
    C. It helps to prevent contact burns on the client's skin.
    D. It prevents skin irritation from the surface of the pack.

Copyright © 2018 Elsevier Canada, a division of Reed Elsevier Canada, Ltd.

MATCHING

Match the types of heat applications with the correct descriptions or statements. The same answer may be used more than once.

25. _____ A moistened soft pad applied over a body area

26. _____ Does not penetrate deeply

27. _____ Temperature must be lower to prevent injury

28. _____ A warm, moist application that involves immersing a body part in heated water

29. _____ The higher temperature needed means burns are still a risk

30. _____ Moist heat is applied to a small area.

31. _____ The water temperature should be hot (36.6° to 41.1°C [97.8° to 105.9°F]).

32. _____ The tub may be used for applying moist heat to a large area.

A. Dry heat

B. Moist heat

C. Compresses

D. Soaks

FILL IN THE BLANKS

33. What happens to blood vessels and blood flow when heat is applied for a long time?

    _____

Copyright © 2018 Elsevier Canada, a division of Reed Elsevier Canada, Ltd.

Working in Acute Care

TRUE OR FALSE

Circle T for true, or circle F for false.

1. **T** **F** A nasal speculum is used to examine the inside of the nose.

2. **T** **F** The lithotomy position is used to examine a client's breasts.

3. **T** **F** You should always weigh your client before an examination.

4. **T** **F** Sims' position is sometimes used to examine the rectum or vagina.

5. **T** **F** The examiner (either the doctor or the nurse) will take all of the specimens to the laboratory.

6. **T** **F** The preoperative period may be many days or just a few minutes.

7. **T** **F** Abdominal surgeries do not usually require a preoperative enema.

8. **T** **F** The support worker is responsible for ensuring that the client's chart is in order before the client goes to the operating room.

9. **T** **F** A thrombus can form in the deep leg veins.

10. **T** **F** Elastic stockings help prevent thrombi.

MULTIPLE RESPONSE

From the list below, choose all of the correct answers.

11. A hospital unit consists of which of the following rooms:
    A. Clean utility room
    B. Nursing station
    C. Pantry (or kitchenette)
    D. Pharmacy
    E. Soiled (dirty) utility room
    F. Apparatus room
    G. Oxygen room
    H. Client rooms

12. What should you explain to the client about the position used during the examination?
    A. Why the position is needed
    B. How to assume the position
    C. How the body is draped for warmth and privacy
    D. What the examiner is looking for
    E. How long the client will stay in the position

Copyright © 2018 Elsevier Canada, a division of Reed Elsevier Canada, Ltd.

13. Which of the following can you do to assist in the psychological care of the surgical client?
    A. Listen to the client voice his or her fears or concerns about surgery.
    B. Answer any questions about the surgery.
    C. Explain to the client procedures you will perform and why they are being done.
    D. Report to your supervisor any verbal and nonverbal signs of client fear and anxiety.
    E. Report to your supervisor the client's request to see a spiritual advisor.

14. Which of the following are fears the client may have about surgery?
    A. Disfigurement and scarring
    B. Disability
    C. Nausea or vomiting
    D. Pain during and after surgery
    E. Dying during surgery
    F. Anaesthesia and its effects
    G. Severe pain or discomfort after surgery
    H. Tubes, needles, and other equipment used for care

15. What valuables should be removed from the client and placed in safekeeping while the client undergoes surgery, if the client has no one to give it to?
    A. Dentures
    B. Glasses
    C. Contact lenses
    D. Lottery tickets
    E. Hearing aid
    F. Cash
    G. Jewellery
    H. Artificial eyes and prostheses

16. How can the support worker protect the client from injury after a preoperative medication has been given?
    A. Have the client walk to the bathroom to void.
    B. Raise bed rails as per hospital policy
    C. Place a lap belt across the client.
    D. Make sure the call bell is within the client's reach.
    E. Place a glass of water next to the client so the client doesn't have to get up.

17. How is the client's room prepared for the client's return from surgery?
    A. Make the bed as a closed bed.
    B. Place a jug of water at the bedside.
    C. Place a kidney basin and tissues at the bedside.
    D. Have the bed in a high-Fowler's position.
    E. Place an IV pole next to the client's bed.

18. Which postoperative observations are important to report to the nurse?
    A. Choking
    B. A drop or rise in blood pressure
    C. Bright red blood from the incision, drainage tubes, or suction tubes
    D. A pulse rate of more than between 80 and 100 beats per minute
    E. A rise or drop in body temperature
    F. Hypoxia
    G. Eupnea
    H. Cold, moist, clammy, or pale skin
    I. The client would like a coffee

19. Which complications can be prevented with early ambulation?
    A. Thrombi
    B. Pneumonia
    C. Atelectasis
    D. Wound pain
    E. Constipation
    F. Emesis
    G. Dehydration

20. Why is it important for the client to be encouraged to deep-breathe and cough after surgery?
    A. It may prevent pneumonia.
    B. It reduces postoperative pain.
    C. It reduces the risk of vomiting.
    D. It promotes urine production.
    E. It reduces the likelihood of lung complications.

Copyright © 2018 Elsevier Canada, a division of Reed Elsevier Canada, Ltd.

MULTIPLE CHOICE

Circle the correct answer.

21. A tuning fork is used to:
    A. Examine the mouth
    B. Examine the inside of the nose
    C. Examine the internal structures of the eye
    D. Test hearing

22. The position the client is usually in for an examination of the abdomen is the:
    A. Lithotomy position
    B. Knee-chest position
    C. Sims' position
    D. Supine position

23. The lithotomy position is used to examine the:
    A. Vagina and perineum
    B. Abdomen
    C. Prostate gland
    D. Chest.

24. Why is a catheter ordered for some surgeries?
    A. To keep the bladder empty during surgery
    B. To prevent bladder infections postoperatively
    C. To prevent incontinence
    D. So that the client does not have to get out of bed to go to the bathroom

25. Why are postoperative leg exercises important for the client to practise?
    A. They help to decrease venous blood flow to the leg.
    B. They help to prevent the formation of a thrombus in the leg.
    C. Exercises reduce hypoxia to the lower leg.
    D. They assist with stabilizing postoperative blood pressure.

26. A general anaesthesia produces:
    A. A loss of sensation or feeling in a large area of the body
    B. Unconsciousness and the loss of feeling or sensation
    C. Loss of sensation in a small area
    D. A partial loss of memory and sensation

27. When a client first returns from the recovery room, how often should vital signs be taken?
    A. Every 15 minutes for the first hour
    B. Every 30 minutes
    C. Every hour for 4 hours
    D. Every 4 hours

MATCHING

Match each description with the correct position.

28. _____ Hips down to edge of table, knees flexed, feet in stirrups

29. _____ Lying on side with upper leg flexed

30. _____ Lying on back with legs together or knees flexed

31. _____ Kneeling with body supported on knees and chest

A. Supine

B. Lithotomy

C. Knee-chest

D. Sims'

Copyright © 2018 Elsevier Canada, a division of Reed Elsevier Canada, Ltd.

Match the descriptions or examples given with the correct type of surgery. The same answer may be used more than once.

32. _____ Done immediately to save the client's life

33. _____ Done when the coronary arteries are blocked

34. _____ Done for the client's well-being

35. _____ Needed after an accident

36. _____ Must be done soon to prevent further damage or disease

37. _____ Cosmetic surgery is an example of this type of surgery

A. Elective surgery

B. Emergency surgery

C. Urgent surgery

Determine when each of these events occurs in relation to the surgical process.

38. _____ Chest X-ray, CBC, and ECG

39. _____ Coughing and deep-breathing exercises as ordered

40. _____ Operative consent must be signed

A. Preoperatively

B. Postoperatively

Copyright © 2018 Elsevier Canada, a division of Reed Elsevier Canada, Ltd.

LABELLING

41. Label each of the examination instruments below.

A. _____

B. _____

C. _____

D. _____

E. _____

F. _____

G. _____

Copyright © 2018 Elsevier Canada, a division of Reed Elsevier Canada, Ltd.

End-of-Life Care

TRUE OR FALSE

Circle T for true, or circle F for false.

1. **T   F**   Many people fear death.

2. **T   F**   During the bargaining stage of grief, the client is usually angry.

3. **T   F**   The client has the right to refuse treatments.

4. **T   F**   As death approaches, the client will need more blankets.

5. **T   F**   Advance directives allow clients to control their future health care.

6. **T   F**   Religious beliefs may help when someone is dying because they can provide comfort.

7. **T   F**   Children younger than 3 years have no concept of death.

8. **T   F**   Children 3–5 years of age know that death is final but may not think that it will happen to them.

9. **T   F**   Listening is an important method of communication when dealing with a dying client.

10. **T   F**   Oral hygiene should be given less frequently as death approaches.

11. **T   F**   When death is near, circulation fails and the pulse is fast, weak, and irregular.

12. **T   F**   The goal of palliative care is to relieve pain and suffering while finding a cure.

13. **T   F**   An advance directive is an informal document in which a person states her wishes about future health care, treatment, and personal care.

14. **T   F**   Mucus collecting in the airway that causes wet gurgling sounds is known as the *death rattle*.

MULTIPLE RESPONSE

From the list below, choose all of the correct answers.

15. How can the support worker help to promote comfort when the dying client has severe pain?
    A. Provide skin care and personal hygiene.
    B. Offer back massages.
    C. Assist with relaxation techniques.
    D. Encourage physical activity.
    E. Keep the person in good body alignment.

Copyright © 2018 Elsevier Canada, a division of Reed Elsevier Canada, Ltd.

16. What rights are protected in the Dying Person's Bill of Rights?
    A. To be treated as a living human being until death
    B. To maintain a sense of hopefulness
    C. To be cared for by those who can maintain a sense of hopefulness
    D. To express feelings and emotions about one's approaching death
    E. To have decisions about one's care made by others
    F. To be free of pain
    G. To die in peace and dignity

17. Some signs of death include the following:
    A. Movement, muscle tone, and sensation are lost.
    B. Peristalsis and other digestive functions slow.
    C. Cheyne–Stokes respirations are common.
    D. Pain increases.
    E. The client usually refuses to eat or drink.

MULTIPLE CHOICE

Circle the correct answer.

18. Which of these beliefs about death is common among young adults?
    A. They may blame themselves when someone dies.
    B. They see death as a reunion with those who have died before them.
    C. They worry about who will care for and support those left behind.
    D. They welcome death as freedom from pain, suffering, and disability.

19. Which of the following statements about providing physical care for a dying client is true?
    A. Sim's position is the best to promote breathing.
    B. The need for repositioning is decreased.
    C. Nutritional needs increase.
    D. Urinary retention and constipation are common.

20. Which of these actions would be helpful to the family of a dying client?
    A. Stay in the room with the family and client as much as possible.
    B. Allow family members to give care.
    C. Ask the family to leave when visiting hours are over.
    D. Ask your clergy member to visit them.

21. Which of a client's rights is violated if a health care worker avoids the dying client?
    A. Right to privacy
    B. Right to confidentiality
    C. Right to be free from abuse, mistreatment, and neglect
    D. Right to protection of personal possessions

22. If a client has a "do not resuscitate" order, what action is appropriate when the client dies?
    A. Begin CPR immediately.
    B. The nurse in charge decides if a code should be called.
    C. The support worker may begin CPR if her own beliefs are opposed to taking no action.
    D. No attempt will be made to resuscitate the client.

23. What is a sign that death is near?
    A. The respiratory system fails.
    B. The body temperature falls.
    C. The pulse rate slows.
    D. Pain increases.

24. Which group of clients has fewer fears about death?
    A. Younger adults
    B. Children
    C. Older adults
    D. Middle-aged adults

25. Which is one of the last functions lost?
    A. Taste
    B. Smell
    C. Hearing
    D. Sight

Copyright © 2018 Elsevier Canada, a division of Reed Elsevier Canada, Ltd.

26. Postmortem care includes:
    A. Repositioning the body
    B. Bathing the body
    C. Removing tubes after permission is given
    D. All of the above

27. A hospice provides:
    A. Palliative care
    B. Active medical care
    C. Care postoperatively
    D. Preoperative care

MATCHING

Match the correct stage of grief with each statement. Note: Answers may be used more than once.

28. _____ The client cannot deal with any problem or decision about his illness.

29. _____ The client may wish to talk about people and things that will be left behind.

30. _____ The client may blame others and be difficult to care for.

31. _____ This stage is done privately and on a spiritual level.

32. _____ The client takes care of unfinished business.

33. _____ The client is sad and mourns things that have been lost.

34. _____ The client refuses to believe death is close.

35. _____ The client may carry on this stage in private.

36. _____ The client may blame others for problems.

37. _____ The client begins to move forward with her life.

A. Denial
B. Anger
C. Bargaining
D. Depression
E. Acceptance

Copyright © 2018 Elsevier Canada, a division of Reed Elsevier Canada, Ltd.

FILL IN THE BLANKS

Recall the Ontario Residents' Bill of Rights (Box 9-2 in Chapter 9), and match the rights of dying clients in long-term care related to the following actions:

A. To have privacy and confidentiality
B. To visit in private with family and friends
C. To be free from abuse, mistreatment, and neglect
D. To be in a safe and homelike setting
E. To maintain personal choice

38. _____ Restraints are used only if ordered by a doctor.

39. _____ Do not expose the client unnecessarily.

40. _____ Try to keep equipment and supplies out of sight.

41. _____ Some people avoid a dying person because of superstitions and religious beliefs.

42. _____ The client may refuse treatment.

43. _____ The client may want certain photographs and religious items nearby.

44. _____ The client's final moments and cause of death are kept confidential.

45. _____ A roommate may have to leave the room if the client is too weak to visit outside the room.

46. _____ The health care team needs to respect the client's choices to refuse treatment and not to prolong life.

47. _____ The client's personal property is protected from loss or damage before and after death.

Copyright © 2018 Elsevier Canada, a division of Reed Elsevier Canada, Ltd.

Starting Your Career

TRUE OR FALSE

Circle T for true, or circle F for false.

1. **T F** The lengthier your resumé, the better it is.

2. **T F** A letter of application is also called a *cover letter.*

3. **T F** Your cover letter should be at least two pages long.

4. **T F** If you email your letter and resumé, it is a good idea to also deliver a hard copy.

5. **T F** If asked, you should tell your prospective employer if you have been fired from a previous job.

6. **T F** When filling out an online job application, you may skip parts that are unimportant to you.

7. **T F** Asking people you know about possible jobs at their workplace is not the best way to find a job.

8. **T F** An employer is not as concerned about your dependability as he or she may be about your job skills.

9. **T F** If you were fired from a previous job, it is all right to write on a job application that you resigned.

10. **T F** When you are being interviewed for a job, it is acceptable to ask about starting salary and vacation time.

MULTIPLE RESPONSE

From the list below, choose all of the correct answers.

11. Main basic resumé styles include:
    A. Chronological resumé: highlights employment history, starting with the most current employment and working backward
    B. Functional resumé: highlights skills or functions and briefly lists positions held
    C. Achievement resumé: highlights all successes and awards earned

12. As you write your resumé, which questions should you ask yourself?
    A. Is the information relevant?
    B. Have I been completely honest?
    C. Have I expressed myself clearly?
    D. Is my resumé consistent?
    E. Is there anything I can leave out?

13. Sources to help you in your job search include:
    A. Employment advertisements on social media sites
    B. Flyers found on windshields
    C. The Internet
    D. College career services
    E. Personal contacts

14. Your letter of application should include:
    A. Relevant skills and qualities
    B. Accomplishments
    C. Contests won
    D. A respectful, capable, and professional tone
    E. Your mailing address

15. In an interview, what is the employer looking for?
    A. Someone with the educational qualifications for the job
    B. Someone who has the skills necessary to do the job or who is able to learn these skills
    C. Someone to whom clients and co-workers will respond well
    D. Someone who is reliable, responsible, and motivated
    E. Someone who is attractive and personable

16. You can prepare for an interview by:
    A. Writing possible answers on cue cards
    B. Making a good impression—paying attention to your grooming and clothing
    C. Practising—focusing on listening skills, relaxation techniques, and responses to questions
    D. Planning—deciding what you are going to wear and the route you will take to get there, and preparing a fresh copy of your resumé
    E. Preparing possible questions and answers

17. You can do several things during the interview to help you get the job. Some of these are:
    A. Use a firm handshake.
    B. Do not use the interviewer's first name.
    C. Project a confident image.
    D. Listen carefully.
    E. Answer questions rapidly.
    F. Answer questions honestly.
    G. Be honest about your previous job even if it was unpleasant.
    H. Use experiences to support opinions.
    I. Ask the right questions.
    J. Thank the interviewer for his or her time.

18. Before accepting a job, find out:
    A. If the offer is conditional
    B. If the job begins with a trial period
    C. If the pay offered is negotiable

19. You have had a job interview and are now planning to write a thank-you note or email to your interviewer. What points should your note include?
    A. You should express your thanks for the interview.
    B. You should show your interest in the position.
    C. You should sign your name.
    D. You should state your impressions about the interviewer.

MULTIPLE CHOICE

Circle the correct answer.

20. When going to an interview, it would be appropriate to:
    A. Have a glass of wine before arriving to relax you.
    B. Wear a sweatsuit and athletic shoes to show that you are physically fit and ready to work.
    C. Avoid wearing heavy perfume or after-shave lotion.
    D. Arrive exactly at the time of the interview so you do not have to wait around in the reception area.

Copyright © 2018 Elsevier Canada, a division of Reed Elsevier Canada, Ltd.

21. Mary Saunders has had four jobs in 1 year. She does not list all four jobs when completing a job application. This is:
    A. Unnecessary information
    B. Invasion of privacy
    C. Deception by omission
    D. Ethically correct

22. You are completing a job application. How many references should you be prepared to give?
    A. One
    B. Two
    C. Three
    D. Four

23. You are in the waiting area before your interview. What should you do?
    A. Text-message your friend on your cellphone.
    B. Talk to the receptionist.
    C. Sit quietly.
    D. File your nails so they look groomed.

24. Which type of answer is best in an interview?
    A. "Yes" and "no" answers
    B. Honest and positive
    C. Long explanations
    D. Count to three and then give a factual answer

25. After a job interview, you should:
    A. Thank the interviewer
    B. State that you look forward to hearing from the interviewer
    C. Shake the interviewer's hand
    D. Do all of the above

26. Why is having a probationary period common practice for new hires?
    A. So the employer can determine if you are the right fit for the job
    B. To prevent new hires from using their benefits
    C. To reduce your stress and anxiety if you are let go
    D. So you don't have to contribute to Canada Pension Plan

Copyright © 2018 Elsevier Canada, a division of Reed Elsevier Canada, Ltd.